OVERDOSE

Also by Benjamin Perrin

Victim Law
Invisible Chains

BENJAMIN PERRIN

OVERDOSE

HEARTBREAK *and* HOPE

in CANADA'S

OPIOID CRISIS

VIKING

VIKING

an imprint of Penguin Canada, a division of Penguin Random House Canada Limited

Canada • USA • UK • Ireland • Australia • New Zealand • India • South Africa • China

First published 2020

LIBRARY AND ARCHIVES CANADA CATALOGUING IN PUBLICATION
Title: Overdose : heartbreak and hope in Canada's opioid crisis / Benjamin Perrin.
Names: Perrin, Benjamin, author.
Identifiers: Canadiana (print) 20190141921 | Canadiana (ebook) 2019014193X | ISBN 9780735237865 (hardcover) | ISBN 9780735237872 (HTML)
Subjects: LCSH: Opioid abuse—Canada. | LCSH: Fentanyl—Canada. | LCSH: Opioids—Overdose. | LCSH: Fentanyl—Overdose—Canada.
Classification: LCC RC568.O45 P47 2020 | DDC 362.29/3—dc23

Book and cover design by Andrew Roberts
Cover image by Julius Reque / Getty Images

Printed and bound in Canada

10 9 8 7 6 5 4 3 2 1

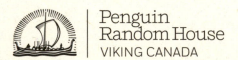

Penguin
Random House
VIKING CANADA

For Douglas "Little Doug" Nickerson

Most people are more comfortable with
old problems than with new solutions.

—*Anonymous*

CONTENTS

FOREWORD

"If they ran a dog as the candidate I'd still vote Conservative."

Growing up in Calgary, I heard that saying more than once. And even though I love dogs and thought of myself as a conservative, it bothered me. It summed up my fears of party politics: at some point, you'd have to shut your mind off and blindly surrender to loyalty and ideology.

I first became interested in politics when I was 14. A federal election had been called for October 25, 1993, and my social studies teacher asked us to keep a scrapbook about it.

I dove into the project. I got copies of each party's election platform and read them voraciously. This was pre-Internet, so I had to clip out newspaper stories with scissors and watch the evening news to learn what each political party leader had said. Even though I couldn't vote, I was fascinated by the tough issues and tried to make up my own mind about them.

In 2012, two decades later and with that election scrapbook sitting in my parents' basement, I found myself at the heart of Canadian politics as Prime Minister Stephen Harper's top criminal justice advisor. I'd taken a one-year leave of absence from my job as a law professor at the University of British Columbia to pursue this once-in-a-lifetime opportunity. I was eager to use my position to help the plight of victims of crime—an area I'd spent most of my professional career working on.

In Harper's office, I also had a front-row seat to Canada's war on drugs. His "tough on crime" agenda had already increased jail time for drug offences and fought unsuccessfully to shut down Insite in Vancouver, at that point the country's only supervised injection site. Since illegal drugs were viewed as bringing disorder and devastation, stamping them out was Conservative dogma. Having never spent much time thinking about drug policy, I figured it made sense. I had shut my mind off.

A few years after moving back to Vancouver with my young family and resuming my job at UBC, I started hearing seemingly isolated media stories about illicit drug overdose deaths in the city. It struck me as a tragic yet senseless loss of life.

As the death toll mounted and a public health emergency was declared in BC in 2016, it was clear that the status quo wasn't working. It bothered me that I was just carrying on with my busy life as people continued to die every day in my city and across the country. I'd been spending time seeking God in dealing with challenges in my own life, so one afternoon I prayed a simple prayer: I asked him to give me a heart of compassion for the people who were being affected by the opioid crisis. I had no idea where it would lead me.

I began asking around the law school to see whether any of my colleagues were conducting research on the opioid crisis. Nope. I checked at the other law schools and posted an appeal on Twitter. It turned out that there wasn't a single law professor in the province—and quite likely the entire country—who was doing any work to address the crisis at the time.

How could I just stand by as people continued to die? I felt a moral responsibility to try to help if I could, and also a personal responsibility to do something. After all, I'd worked for a government that set up

Canada's current approach to dealing with illegal drugs—a modern-day war on drugs—and it was clearly failing to address this crisis. I was a law professor with experience in government and had helped change laws and policies before. I had contacts in law enforcement and the community. I knew how to get a message out through the media and had contacts with a major publisher. And with tenure, I could take controversial positions based on my research. It was time to act.

I set out to investigate the opioid crisis without any team or funding in place. That would come later. It was a leap of faith. My aim was to find out why the crisis was happening, what was being done about it, and what more could be done to save lives. I would follow the trail of evidence wherever it led.

I dropped everything to kick-start my research. And given that this was a public health emergency, I didn't want to wait a year or two to apply for traditional research grants; instead, I proposed raising the money I'd need via crowdfunding. The law school put the brakes on that idea. Fortunately, an individual donor stepped up to cover the costs of a research assistant, travel, and transcription services for the interviews I needed to do.

Within a month or two I'd read all the current reports on the problem and gotten ethics approval to launch the study. Then I hit the streets. I quickly learned that BC is the epicentre of the opioid crisis in Canada, and that Vancouver, Surrey, and Victoria have been hardest hit. So that's where I focused my investigation.

I interviewed 42 leading experts with over 500 years of combined professional experience. I met with police chiefs, drug squad investigators, undercover police agents, border guards, intelligence analysts, firefighters, prosecutors, defence lawyers, judges, healthcare officials, medical doctors, addiction specialists, community-based service organizations, Indigenous organizations, activists, advocates, and organizations representing people who use drugs.

I criss-crossed the BC Lower Mainland and travelled to Victoria to see firsthand what was happening. I filed Freedom of Information requests to get access to government records. I analyzed and wrote up my findings as soon as I received interview transcripts back, working from early in the morning, before the kids were awake, to late into the night. Burning the midnight oil, I felt like I was back in law school again, except now I needed to take a 15-minute nap in the afternoon.

I was looking for answers to the tough questions I had, questions I kept hearing every time the opioid crisis seemed to pop up in conversation:

- What is the opioid crisis?
- Why is fentanyl killing so many people?
- Why do people start using? Why can't they stop?
- Has criminalizing drugs failed?
- Why are dealers killing their customers?
- Can we stop fentanyl at its source?
- Who's been hardest hit?
- Can we prosecute our way out?
- What is naloxone and is it the solution?
- Don't supervised injection sites enable drug use?
- Is providing "safe drugs" giving up on people?
- How can we help people stop using?
- Won't decriminalization make things worse?
- How can we solve this crisis?

By the end of my intensive 100-day investigation, I'd made a complete 180-degree turn. I was convinced: the misguided war on drugs was not only a total failure, it was actually making things worse. The casualties of this war include the thousands who've died from illicit drug overdoses, most often dying alone because of the stigma that flows in large part from criminalization. Their suffering was invisible to most of us. They were counted only as they died. And unless something radical is done today, countless more of our neighbours, friends, and loved ones risk the same fate.

This book is a chronicle of my investigation into the opioid crisis. It's a story about lives lost and people saved. It's a story of heartbreak and hope—a raw, tragically real story that I never expected to write but felt compelled to set down. For me, it's also part of my story of personal transformation, a change of mind and of heart.

— 1 —

WHAT IS THE OPIOID CRISIS?

I don't think anybody really saw this coming.
—*Dr. Mark Tyndall, Executive Director, BC Centre for Disease Control*

A sleepy suburb on the outskirts of Greater Vancouver was about to get a wake-up call—in more ways than one. At 1:30 a.m., the stillness of a balmy late-summer night in Delta was shattered by the blaring siren and flashing lights of an ambulance racing to a family home.

"The paramedic walked up to a house in Delta because a friend of somebody called 911 saying this guy's passed out; he's not breathing," said Linda Lupini, who heads BC Emergency Health Services. "Before they got into the house there were two kids who'd overdosed on the front stairs. So they thought they were at the address—the kids are overdosed; that's the call."

The paramedics began working frantically to help resuscitate them. The tell-tale signs of a drug overdose include unresponsiveness, blue lips, and difficulty breathing—or not breathing at all. The outcome can be fatal.

"Are you coming upstairs?!" someone screamed from inside the house.

"What do you mean?" replied a confused paramedic.

"The kid we called for is upstairs."

There were three simultaneous drug overdoses at the house that night—and that was just the beginning. Within 26 minutes the 911 switchboard lit up like a Christmas tree. Drug overdose calls kept coming in. Paramedics would revive someone only to learn from them that someone else had taken drugs at the same party and could be at risk.

"Then we were working with dispatch, trying to find all these kids," said Lupini.

In total, 11 young people who were at the party overdosed the night of September 1, 2016, after taking what they thought was a small amount of cocaine. What they didn't know was that it had been laced with fentanyl—a potent opioid drug. One went into full cardiac arrest.

"We had parents doing CPR on the front lawn on their kids," said Lupini. "We had 11 teenagers literally not breathing. They were all resuscitated, but barely. A few came close to not making it. It was so traumatic for the front-line staff. We just didn't have the resources to respond to something like that.

"The problem for an ambulance service is that the increase in calls are your highest acuity—Code 3," she continued. "They're gonna die in minutes."

———

Between January 2016 and June 2019, a record-shattering 13,913 people across Canada died from opioid-related drug overdoses. In 2018, when the annual death count hit 4588, a life was lost every two hours. According to Dr. Theresa Tam, Canada's chief public health officer, opioid-related overdoses have become the leading cause of death for 30- to 39-year-olds. And although every part of the country has been affected by the opioid crisis, British Columbia, Alberta, Ontario, Saskatchewan, and Manitoba have been the hardest hit.

On April 14, 2016, British Columbia declared the opioid crisis a public health emergency after illicit drug overdose deaths began sky-rocketing. Historically, about 200 to 300 people a year had lost their lives this way, but by 2015 the number of overdose deaths had risen to 530. Worst was yet to come. By 2018 that number had almost tripled, reaching 1542. It hit me just how serious the situation was when the BC Coroners Service announced that illicit drugs were claiming more lives than murder, suicide, and car accidents combined. By 2019, the number of overdose deaths in the province finally started to decline as thousands had already died and the response to the crisis ramped out, even as the number of 911 overdose calls continued to grow to almost 25,000.

"For the longest while we said it's a crisis," said Jennifer Breakspear, executive director of the Portland Hotel Society (PHS) Community Services Society, which provides supportive housing for over 2000 people in Vancouver and Victoria as well as various programs and services. PHS also operates Insite, North America's first supervised injection site. Breakspear was hired to head up PHS in January 2017. And although she'd had experience in leading a non-profit focused on reproductive health, she described the transition to PHS as a real "crash course."

As I sat on a couch in Breakspear's office on East Hastings Street, fire truck and ambulance sirens kept interrupting her—a constant reminder that Vancouver's Downtown Eastside is ground zero in this crisis. "The soundtrack of my workday," she remarked as another emergency vehicle raced by. Without a doubt, several of them that hour would have been heading to overdoses in the immediate area.

When the public health emergency was declared in 2016, Breakspear told me, everyone thought it was the height of the crisis. Since then, though, "the numbers have continued to worsen. I don't want to say it's become the normal—the new norm. That sounds so offensive," she said. "This is still a situation in which people are dying every day, and I don't know how you could ever wrap your head around calling it 'normal.'"

That harsh realization is especially disturbing for the loved ones of those who've died during this overdose crisis. "The thought that it's the new normal is just crushing," said Leslie McBain, co-founder of Moms Stop the Harm, a national advocacy group of families that have lost loved ones to drug overdoses, including her own son. "Fentanyl is still out there; it's still killing people. People have no alternative."

"Crisis" is the word that everyone I spoke to used to describe this state of affairs, including police officers, medical experts, and groups of people who use drugs alike. And BC is like the canary in a coal mine; the problem has spread across the rest of the country, too. The only place you'd see more body bags would be in an actual war. But even that's not an entirely accurate comparison: 159 courageous Canadians died during the conflict in Afghanistan, and 516 died during the Korean War. Combined, those losses are significantly lower than the number of Canadians who died from fatal overdoses in 2018 alone.

Given the massive fatalities during the opioid crisis, Vancouver's morgue has been filled to capacity and the BC Coroners Service has been forced to develop extraordinary plans to store bodies while the coroner investigates. "We are in urgent need of temporary body storage owing to the public health emergency," wrote Aaron Burns with the BC Ministry of Justice in a December 19, 2016, email plea to funeral home directors in the BC Lower Mainland. (The email was released under the Freedom of Information and Protection of Privacy Act.) "Bodies are kept at hospital morgues or funeral homes while the coroner conducts the investigation," Burns continued. "It would only be situations where those places are overwhelmed by volume that storage would pose a problem for us. That being said, we've come close to that point in the recent past and looked into refrigerated shipping containers as a contingency."

The impact of the opioid crisis is widespread. For people who use drugs, it means never knowing whether they'll be next. It means being blamed. It means being treated like criminals and lowlifes. This crisis continues to catastrophically affect families, friends, and loved ones of those who have died or are using substances and are at risk. And it's had a devastating impact on those working hard to save lives, including "peers"—people with lived experience using drugs—and professional first responders like paramedics, firefighters, and police officers.

Carolyn Sinclair is the manager of the BC Provincial Overdose Mobile Response Team, which provides crisis support to professional first responders. I first met Sinclair several years ago in her previous role as head of Police Victim Services of BC. She knows about supporting people in traumatic situations and she knows law enforcement. That, combined with her positive outlook and cheerful attitude, made her the perfect person for this new job. Her team was set up when it became clear that the relentless trauma of the opioid crisis was hitting first responders hard.

"In April 2018 we had 27 completed suicides by first responders," said Sinclair. It was a startling figure, one that she believes is directly linked to the opioid crisis. I asked her to tell me about some of these individuals so that I could get a better idea of how this public health emergency was affecting them. In one instance, she said, "the firefighters arrived at the house and found a mom down. The first person in was a young firefighter. They didn't realize that there was a little four-year-old girl that had also gotten into Mom's drugs and that she'd crawled behind a chair. They didn't know she was there until later. The little girl is still in an induced coma, and there are some firefighters that are visiting her every day. The first firefighter to that scene committed suicide."

———

The opioid epidemic has spread across the continent like wildfire. In the United States, more than 500,000 people died from drug overdoses between 2000 and 2015. And those figures have been accelerating, as they've been in Canada, owing to a dramatic increase in synthetic opioid–related deaths. In 2017, an estimated 70,237 people died from illicit drug overdoses in the U.S. That's more than the total number of American troops, 58,220, who died between 1961 and 1975 during the entire Vietnam War.

In response, on October 26, 2017, the United States declared the opioid crisis a national public health emergency. Canada has yet to take that step. But despite the U.S. declaration, even the most rudimentary medical interventions that have been proven to save lives (such as "take-home" naloxone—the antidote to an opioid overdose—and supervised consumption sites) have faced roadblocks. President Donald Trump has instead insisted on building a wall on the US–Mexico border to deal with the problem—an idea that experts agree would do nothing to address it.

What's responsible for causing this carnage?

The opioid crisis has many complex and interrelated causes. But the immediate starting point is a drug I'd never heard of until it started popping up in news reports about overdose deaths: fentanyl.

"The main driver of the crisis that we're in is the contaminated drug supply, and we have little to no control over it," said Chris Buchner, director of communicable diseases and harm reduction at Fraser Health, which covers the sprawling suburbs outside of Vancouver and has the unfortunate distinction of having the highest number of illicit drug overdose deaths of any health authority in the province.

"It's horrendous. I hate people calling it 'overdose,' because people are being poisoned. 'Overdose' means they used too much. They're using what they normally would," said Shelda Kastor with the Western Aboriginal Harm Reduction Society. Indeed, Kastor's explanation is backed up by data from the coroner's office.

In 2012, fentanyl was found in just 4% of post-mortem toxicology investigations of illicit drug overdose deaths in BC—a negligible amount that no one really paid much attention to. Since then, illicit drug overdose deaths where fentanyl has been detected (on its own or combined with other drugs, such as cocaine, methamphetamine, and heroin) jumped to 15% in 2013, 25% in 2014, 29% in 2015, 67% in 2016, 82% in 2017, and a staggering 87% in 2018. Multiple drug use, including alcohol, is frequently identified in these cases, with fentanyl as a common denominator.

When you look at the annual number of illicit drug overdose deaths over the last decade—taking out those where fentanyl was detected—you see a relatively stable rate. In 2007 and 2017 alike, there were roughly 200 illicit drug overdose deaths in BC that did not involve fentanyl. Illicit fentanyl is clearly the immediate cause of the dramatic rise in overdose deaths. But, as I would find out, there was plenty of blame to be shared for this crisis.

– 2 –

WHY IS FENTANYL
KILLING SO MANY PEOPLE?

"I don't have to breathe."

That's the thought that passed through Laurence Rankin's mind as fentanyl began to cause him respiratory depression.

"Breathe. Don't forget to breathe," the nurse reminded Rankin, who was recovering from surgery in the hospital and had been given fentanyl to relieve the pain.

As deputy chief constable of the Vancouver Police Department, Rankin oversees the force's response to the opioid crisis. His experience in the hospital helped him understand some of what's going on when a person overdoses from illicit fentanyl. Fortunately for Rankin, who'd been given precisely titrated quantities of the potent painkiller and under medical supervision, he was fine. Illicit fentanyl has neither of those safeguards.

Canada's illicit drug supply is contaminated. Experts say that fentanyl has been found in all street drugs except cannabis (contrary to some erroneous media reports), and that it has saturated the illicit opioid market. What's sold as heroin in Vancouver often contains little, if any, pure white heroin. Instead, it's a toxic cocktail that can consist of nothing more than "buffers," like table salt and caffeine, with a few grains of fentanyl mixed in.

"The drug supply is shifting rapidly," said Dr. Evan Wood, executive director of the BC Centre on Substance Use and a practising physician. "In clinic, we would see people and tell them that their urine toxicology screen had fentanyl, and they'd be surprised because they thought they were using other opioids, like heroin or OxyContin [a synthetic opioid pain-relief medication]."

Pure fentanyl comes in the form of tiny crystals or a white powder. Mixed into other substances, it's invisible to the naked eye, odourless, and tasteless. There's no way to tell whether a substance contains fentanyl without testing it. And even then you won't know how much of the drug is mixed in.

"As long as we're asking people every day to play Russian roulette with these drugs, people are going to continue to die," said Dr. Mark Tyndall with the BC Centre for Disease Control.

———

What *is* fentanyl, exactly? It's a synthetic opioid, meaning that it's not naturally occurring. Rather, it's made through a chemical process—and, as a result, it has a potentially limitless supply.

"Fentanyl was originally developed for palliative cancer patients, and then it started to be used in some other kinds of pain management," explained Linda Lupini, executive vice president of the BC Provincial Health Services Authority and BC Emergency Health Services. We were sitting in her seventh-floor office in downtown Vancouver. Lupini has thick, black-rimmed glasses and short dark hair. She was eager to help me understand the scope of the problem. Her experience with the opioid crisis is invaluable, as she's run the province-wide ambulance service since 2014. Her team of analysts figured out that there was an epidemic of illicit drug overdoses, and they alerted the BC Ministry of Health back in 2015—the year before the public health emergency was declared. The team, which rapidly deploys resources to respond to clusters of overdoses, has had to develop innovative ways to reach vulnerable people. Every morning when she wakes up, Lupini told me, she checks her phone to see how many overdose calls and deaths there were the night before. It sounded like a horrible way to start the day.

Fentanyl's intended medical purpose is as a powerful painkiller, sedative, and anaesthetic. A key feature is its potency: fentanyl is 30 to 50 times more potent than heroin and 50 to 100 times more potent than morphine. For most people, as little as two milligrams of fentanyl is a lethal dose. How small is that? Imagine just a few grains of table salt.

How exactly does a fentanyl overdose kill someone?

"Fentanyl turns off the receptors that make you breathe," said Lupini. "They slowly turn them off and you just literally go to sleep, but then you stop breathing in your sleep and you're dead, essentially."

It surprised me when I learned that fentanyl isn't a new drug. In fact, it was invented in 1959 by Dr. Paul Janssen, a Belgian physician; in the 1960s it began to be used to treat people in medical settings as well as animals in veterinary medicine.

I was curious about when fentanyl made the leap to being used as an illicit narcotic outside these legal settings, so I did some case law research to see when it first made it onto the radar of the criminal justice system. It turns out that a veterinary office in Beauharnois, Quebec, just south of Montreal on the St. Lawrence River, was the unlikely location of Canada's first reported fentanyl trafficking case. On October 17, 1980, Dr. Jules Blanchette, a 36-year-old veterinary surgeon, sold Inovar-Vet—an anaesthetic for animals containing fentanyl—for $200 to an undercover RCMP officer.

Blanchette also purchased 63 grams of cocaine from a pharmacist he knew for resale on the black market. Blanchette was convicted.

The first time fentanyl is mentioned in any reported judicial decisions as being mixed or cut into street drugs was in a 2008 decision in Nova Scotia, where an expert identified fentanyl as one of a long list of illicit drugs that had been found in what was being sold as Ecstasy pills. So there's some evidence of at least experimental diversion of licit fentanyl dating back almost 40 years and fentanyl being cut into street drugs over a decade ago. However, illicit fentanyl in street drugs doesn't appear to have become widespread in the drug supply in BC until 2012–2013.

Dr. Janssen, who invented fentanyl, died in 2003, while he was attending a scientific conference in Rome. He never lived to experience the bitter irony that the drug he'd created to alleviate pain and suffering would ultimately bring so much misery and death.

If fentanyl sounds formidable, even more potent illicit drugs are now being detected in post-mortem exams. Carfentanyl is a chemical variation, or "analogue," of fentanyl that was never intended for human consumption; it's used in extremely small doses to sedate large animals like elephants. (In the movie *Jurassic World*, carfentanyl is used to sedate a Tyrannosaurus rex.) Carfentanyl is 100 times more potent than fentanyl and 10,000 times more potent than morphine. In fact, it's so powerful that security experts are concerned that terrorist groups could use it in aerosol form as a weapon of mass destruction.

We don't yet know how long carfentanyl has been part of the opioid crisis, since the BC Coroners Service started standard toxicology testing for it only in June 2017. Prior to that, it would have simply been identified as fentanyl. But since then, in just 10 months carfentanyl was detected in 81 illicit drug overdose deaths in BC. A batch of street drugs containing the substance is what keeps first responders up at night. Remarkably, though, some people, likely long-term drug users, are consuming it and surviving. They've developed a tolerance to it. "What's amazing is the degree of carfentanyl positivity in living men that are giving urine drug screens that are getting analyzed," said Dr. Wood. "You see 20% of fentanyl-positive samples that are actually carfentanyl positive."

———

But how did we end up with illicit fentanyl becoming so widespread in street drugs?

"The current situation is very scary," said Oren Bick, senior counsel with the Public Prosecution Service of Canada. "I don't know if it has an end. I think it's a continuation of a historical cat-and-mouse game where people who want to sell narcotics, controlled substances, continue to find more unusual, more innovative ways of doing it."

Bick is an experienced federal drug prosecutor. I first met him over 15 years ago when we were law students at the University of Toronto. He was friendly, bright, and the kind of guy who'd happily share his notes with you if you missed a lecture. Bick and I would occasionally discuss cases from our criminal law class, sometimes over a beer or two. Unlike me, he didn't seem to have aged at all in the intervening years. I'd seen his name in the media as the lead prosecutor on a big fentanyl trafficking case, so I'd decided to reconnect with him.

"Every action has an equal and opposite reaction," said Bick, explaining why illicit fentanyl started to become widespread around 2012. Back then, the big concern in Ottawa was prescription drug abuse. A growing number of pharmaceutical opioids were being misused, and an increasing number were finding their way onto the streets. The knee-jerk solution was to crack down on those drugs. It seemed to make sense at the time.

Most notoriously, OxyContin was widely available in the black market. It was being crushed, mixed with water, and then injected by people who use intravenous drugs as an alternative to illicit opioids like heroin. In 2012, the drug manufacturer responded by transforming OxyContin into a different drug, OxyNeo, which was designed to be "tamper-resistant": it reportedly turned to a flat pancake when crushed and into a gel when it got wet, making it much harder to inject.

But that transformation had its own effects. "When you have this crisis of people abusing OxyContin and the response is to change the formulation of OxyContin to OxyNeo, which is supposedly less susceptible to abuse, enterprising drug dealers find a way to address that by manufacturing their own OxyContin out of fentanyl, with little regard to the consequences, obviously," Bick told me. "Then when that's so financially successful, they start to realize, 'Hey, why are we even selling heroin anymore? Why on earth are we risking our necks to bring heroin in from Asia when we can get fentanyl so much easier, so much cheaper, and make our own heroin?' So once the OxyContin opening hit, that made people understand that fentanyl could be used as a substitute for other opiates. There was no going back."

Bick's explanation of the tectonic shift that's taken place since 2012 in the illicit drug market represents quite a paradox. The attempt to crack down on prescription drug abuse had backfired, and it was this unintended consequence that prosecutors, police, and groups that represent people who use drugs all pointed to as one of the main catalysts for the current crisis.

"The government had no exit strategy once they took OxyContin off the market," said Jordan Westfall, president of the Canadian Association of People Who Use Drugs. "Those people still needed to use drugs. Watching this happen, it's traumatic, it's horrific. It just confirms that this whole approach is not working."

———

I wanted to know what role, if any, the alleged overprescription of opioids by doctors has played in the opioid crisis. In the United States, there's strong evidence that in recent years it has directly and indirectly contributed to an increasing number of overdose deaths. As a result, there have even been criminal charges against doctors in the U.S. and lawsuits against pharmaceutical companies.

"To some extent the medical profession has brought this upon us by not very responsible prescribing, and the pharmaceutical industry by overselling and misleading," said Dr. Richard Frank, a professor of health economics at Harvard. Dr. Frank worked in President Barack Obama's administration coordinating the Department of Health & Human Services' response to the opioid epidemic.

Purdue Pharma introduced OxyContin in the mid-1990s, claiming that its delayed absorption was "believed to reduce the abuse liability"; in other words, allegedly suggesting that it was less addictive. Physicians were allegedly the target of aggressive marketing, including OxyContin-branded swag like fishing hats and stuffed toys, along with "starter coupons" that would give patients a free initial supply of the opioid medication. Medical residents were allegedly taught that, if the patient was in true pain, they didn't need to worry about the potential for addiction. Opioid prescription rates skyrocketed, with drug overdose deaths in the United States steadily increasing from 1999 to 2012. And since then, as illicit fentanyl became widespread, there has been an even greater increase in drug overdose deaths.

In February 2018, after making more than US$35 billion from selling OxyContin, Purdue Pharma announced that it would no longer market opioids to doctors in the United States and that it was cutting its sales force in half. The company has denied deceptive marketing in numerous lawsuits brought against it. In September 2019, the company filed for bankruptcy due to a growing number of lawsuits for its alleged role in the opioid crisis.

"The fact is that we are awash with more opioid pills than we need," said Dr. Frank, "and, at least in the United States, [for] most people who wind up misusing pain medication, the prescription typically wasn't for them. It was for somebody else. We're just allowing a lot of extras to be floating around, which then creates this secondary market."

In central and eastern Canada, there appears to be a clear link to pharmaceutical products playing a role in the black market, particularly fentanyl patches prescribed for pain management. Those patches have been cut up and have made their way onto the illicit market, leading to requirements that patients return used patches before getting another one from their pharmacist. Some people have even chewed used fentanyl patches, trying to suck out that last bit of fentanyl.

A CBC investigation found that an average of half a million doses of prescription drugs are stolen every year from pharmacies, and that the majority of these are opioids. Prescription drug theft has been increasing in provinces like Ontario, but has substantially declined in BC since 2012. Indeed, all the BC-based experts I interviewed agreed that there isn't any noticeable quantity of prescription fentanyl products being diverted to the black market. Some pointed to a study by the BC Coroners Service which found that relatively few overdose deaths—about 75 annually—are caused directly by prescribed opioids.

But what about the indirect role of overprescribing opioids? You know, the stories we've all heard about: a doctor prescribes opioids to a patient who becomes addicted, then cuts the patient off, forcing the patient to seek out dangerous street drugs. That's where I heard some different views.

"I'm sure you could find testimonials in a lot of newspapers of a person who had a leg injury and then their doctor gave them drugs and they liked the drugs and now they continue with drugs and now they're living in the Downtown Eastside," said Dr. Mark Tyndall. "I mean there are potential stories about that, but it's highly unusual, and [with] most of those people, there's probably other factors involved in why they ended up that way."

But other medical experts I talked to in BC weren't quite as categorical.

"We hear a lot in the media about people becoming prescription opioid addicted initially—and there's a case in the Victoria *Times Colonist* newspaper this weekend of a young person, a high school student I think was 16 years old, who had multiple surgeries in the last year and then became prescription opioid addicted," said Dr. Evan Wood. "Then, as they're not able to get prescription opioids, turning to other drug use. So there's that pathway for sure. I think that's very common in the United States, where the overprescription of opioids was a huge issue. Canada is number two in the world, second only after the States in terms of prescription opiate prescribing. So there's certainly that pattern of use."

The news story that Dr. Wood was talking about concerned 16-year-old Elliot Eurchuk, who'd been injured playing sports and underwent four surgeries for sports-related injuries. Against his parents' wishes, Elliot was prescribed opioids for the pain. They were reportedly told that he was old enough to make his own treatment decisions. Elliot was subsequently expelled from high school for using drugs. On the morning of April 20, 2018, his parents found him in his bedroom; tragically, he had died from a drug overdose. The BC Coroners Service is investigating his death.

"Then there's the pattern of use where people become addicted to street opioids, whether that be counterfeit pills, heroin, fentanyl, or other opioids that people are becoming addicted to on the streets," said Dr. Wood. "I think it's multifactorial, but they're certainly the two big pathways I think are getting people addicted."

Preliminary data from a study by the BC Centre for Disease Control found that people who overdosed were more likely to have been on long-term prescribed opioids for pain than the average person, but that at the time of their illicit drug overdose most did not have an active prescription. Indeed, people who use drugs and activists are adamant that some doctors are contributing to the opioid crisis by cutting off people who've become addicted to prescribed opioids and who then end up turning to street drugs.

"We've been sitting with people who, a year ago, had a home. They got cut off their prescriptions and went to the illicit market and have now faced I can't even remember how many overdoses just in a matter of months," said a representative of Pivot Legal Society, a legal advocacy organization that's litigated cases all the way to the Supreme Court of Canada. "And they're now in the criminal justice system—someone who is struggling with cancer, was cut off his pain medication, and is now using on the illicit market. These are extremely real things."

"The drug manufacturers—some of their practices in pushing this stuff to people were exploitative and very aggressive," said Westfall, who himself used illicit opioids for several years and now represents thousands of people who use drugs across Canada.

There's been a big push for doctors to tighten up their prescribing practices around opioids. Studies have also come out recently that question whether less addictive alternatives could do an equal job of providing pain relief. That may make sense for people who aren't yet addicted to opioids, prescribed or otherwise. But what about those who are already using prescribed opioids and have become addicted? A blunt crackdown on them could backfire, running the obvious risk that those patients may resort to toxic street drugs instead.

"Pharmaceutical drugs are sort of drying up," said Westfall. "More people are just turning to fentanyl or street heroin." As surprising as his claim was to me, I would soon learn that the opioid crisis was affecting people from all walks of life—including those whom you'd least expect to use illicit drugs.

— 3 —

WHY DO PEOPLE START USING?
WHY CAN'T THEY STOP?

Buddhist teacher, yoga instructor, father, opioid user.

To the outside world, Michael Stone was the last person you'd think would become a casualty in the opioid crisis. The renowned Zen Buddhist teacher and charismatic yoga instructor led retreats and workshops across Canada and internationally. He spoke at TEDx Toronto and authored books like *Yoga for a World Out of Balance* and *Freeing the Body, Freeing the Mind*. He even created a guided meditation app.

"The majority of people who study with me don't consider themselves to be spiritual," wrote Michael. "I help them decrease stress and anxiety, decrease reactivity, quiet the mind, increase contentment, foster embodiment, live healthily, and to enjoy well-being."

The forty-two-year-old lived with his wife, Carina, and their two children on idyllic Pender Island in British Columbia's picturesque Southern Gulf Islands. He had a child from another relationship as well. Michael also lived with bipolar disorder. Although he'd experimented with psychedelic drugs in his teens and early twenties, he instead came to rely on his practice and self-care for relief: meditation, exercise, early to bed, special diets. He was getting help from naturopaths, herbalists, personal trainers, and therapists. However, as things became increasingly difficult for him to manage, he sought help from a psychiatrist and eventually went on medication. When that didn't seem enough to stabilize him, the prescribed dosage was increased.

"Now and then he would mention a wish for a safe, non-addictive prescribed natural form of opium," explained Carina. "He thought it might calm his overactive mind. Unbeknownst to everybody, he was growing more desperate."

Carina was pregnant with their third child on July 13, 2017, when Michael left for a quick, routine trip to Victoria on nearby Vancouver Island. He never returned home. Using his cell phone call log, Michael's family has tried to piece together what happened on his last day.

"On the way into town he called a substance abuse and addictions pharmacy, likely to ask for a safe, controlled drug to self-medicate. He was not a candidate. He got a haircut, exercised, ran household errands, and finally acquired a street drug."

When Michael didn't return home that night, Carina called the RCMP to file a missing person report. Around midnight, the police found Michael unconscious in his vehicle. Paramedics administered multiple doses of naloxone and intubated him. He was pronounced dead at 1:30 a.m. The coroner's investigation found that he'd died of acute fentanyl toxicity caused by an unintentional illicit substance overdose. He was kept on life support for two more days, with Carina at his bedside, so that his organs could be donated.

Out of this tragedy, his children were left without a dad and Carina was widowed, but three other people got a new lease on life because of Michael's organ donation. A week after his death, a GoFundMe page was launched to support Carina and her children, raising over $130,000.

"It may be hard to put one's mind into his, to imagine how he could take such a risk with a young family, baby on the way, with such a full life and such fortune. Rather than feel the shame and tragedy of it, can we find questions? What was he feeling? How was he coping?

"What can we do for ourselves and others who have impulses or behaviours we cannot understand? Impulses that scare us and silence us? How can we take care of each other?" asked Carina.

———

Michael Stone is one of thousands of people who have died from illicit drug overdoses. Each of them has left friends, family, and loved ones behind. Who exactly is using illicit opioids, and why?

"It's across the board," said Leslie McBain, co-founder of Moms Stop the Harm. "[From] families in poverty and traumatized and their kids end up on the Downtown Eastside to every single socioeconomic strata there is. There's the families of professionals, the lawyers, the doctors. People that are living in communities all across Canada. It can be anyone's child. It's in every corner."

In BC, the vast majority of illicit drug overdose deaths are men (82%), and 90% of victims were between 19 and 59 years old (with 30- to 49-year-olds disproportionately affected). Of those who have recently died from an illicit drug overdose, 80% had a pattern of daily or regular illicit drug use; 9% used illicit drugs occasionally (on weekends or once a month); and 1% had no evidence of illicit drug use in the last year. In the remainder of cases it wasn't possible to determine the frequency of drug use.

———

Where are these overdose deaths happening?

"People are dying primarily because they've been using substances indoors, using alone, often unable to summon help because if they're using alone they don't have somebody there to administer naloxone or call 911 if they get a bad batch," said Andy Watson with the BC Coroners Service. "Really, this is driving home the fact that we have a toxic drug supply."

Data from the Coroners Service defies the popular myth that the overdose crisis is exclusively about homeless street-drug users overdosing in places like Vancouver's Downtown Eastside: only 9% of illicit drug overdose deaths were officially homeless people. Still, many other overdose deaths also occurred in such precarious housing locations as shelters and single room occupancy (SRO) facilities. As a result, much of the response to the opioid crisis has been targeted to these impoverished areas, leading to significant improvements in rates of surviving an overdose. According to Vancouver Fire Chief Darrell Reid, if someone overdoses from illicit drugs in a private residence outside of Vancouver's Downtown Eastside, their chances of dying are three times greater than if they overdosed within that area.

In BC in 2017, 59% of illicit drug overdose deaths occurred in private residences, 25% in other residences (e.g., hotels, motels, rooming houses, shelters), 12% outdoors (e.g., streets, vehicles, sidewalks, parking lots, public parks, wooded areas), and the remainder of cases in other locations, such as inside public buildings and businesses. More than half (52%) of illicit drug overdose deaths involved people using alone, and that number is rising.

"I think many people didn't realize the extent to which broad segments of the population were using illicit opioids, but now we know about it, because we see them dying and it's really challenging to get control of it," said Chris Buchner with Fraser Health.

Buchner was an HIV/AIDS activist in the 1980s and 1990s. He earned his social work degree and then a master's degree in health administration. He's been at the forefront of efforts in BC to stop the spread of communicable diseases and reduce the health risks faced by people who use drugs. And although Buchner helps lead the health authority's response to the opioid crisis from within the system, his urgency and tone showed me that he hasn't lost the voice of a passionate advocate. That's just what is needed most right now.

"There are a large number of people who are employed, have stable lives, relatively stable housing situations, [but] who are dependent on illegal opioids," explained Buchner. "That didn't become noticeable because, you know, [with] opioids, if they're not poisoned and people can predict and understand what's there, the worst thing that can often typically happen to someone is that they get constipated or they get drowsy."

However, with an inconsistently tainted street drug supply, people don't know what they're getting, or its potency. That results in a greater risk of an overdose, which can be fatal if the person is using alone or the people that they're with don't know what to do. So why are so many people using illicit drugs alone, where the risk of dying from an overdose is so much greater?

"The big challenge now is stigma," said Dr. Bonnie Henry, BC's chief medical officer, whose predecessor declared the opioid crisis a public health emergency. "People are using alone, and most of them, they have family, they have friends who often don't even know what they're using, and so it's all about shame and about stigma and about how to have conversations.

"This is not 'those addicts,'" she continued. "This is your brother, your uncle, your sister, your mother, and father. You think about why people use street drugs, and a lot of it has to do with pain, whether it's psychological, emotional, or physical pain that gets people into it." (Two other reasons focus groups have found for why illicit drug users are using alone are their belief that they can "handle it" by themselves and an unwillingness to share their drugs.)

"It could be your neighbour," said Dr. Ronald Joe, medical director for substance use services at Vancouver Coastal Health. "They're occurring throughout Vancouver. The initial indicators are that this is a group that's isolated, socially isolated, who don't have or who have difficulty in accessing healthcare services. Many have concurrent mental health issues. So [these are] people who don't feel they can reach out for help."

"This is highly prevalent in different areas in society and now across socioeconomic boundaries, more than I think at least historical views and presumptions would lead us to believe," said Dr. Evan Wood.

In terms of professions, some experts have identified young men working in the trades as a group that's seen a sizable share of illicit opioid overdose deaths. "Stereotypically, if you're a male between the ages of 20 and 35 and you work in the trades industry and you've suffered an injury and you're no longer on prescription meds, you have a higher risk of using fentanyl," said Dwayne McDonald, assistant commissioner and officer in charge of the RCMP Surrey detachment. "We've seen that."

"We identified that the trades were disproportionately represented in terms of overdoses and overdose deaths," said Buchner's colleague Dr. Aamir Bharmal, who is the medical health officer and medical director of communicable diseases and harm reduction with Fraser Health. "I think it's the fact that the trades are a large employer. We know that the trades employ a lot of men who are younger and potentially within this age demographic category. Then there's also those pieces around the injury and potentially that pathway as well."

Dr. Paul Hasselback, a medical health officer for central Vancouver Island, has another view: "We tend to see an overrepresentation of occupations that don't require criminal record checks. They're long-term, experienced users," he told me. It seems the jury is still out on the reasons why the trades are coming up more often in overdose death statistics.

I was surprised to learn about another group of people who are turning to illicit drugs: professional first responders, including police officers and paramedics.

"Those first responders that have had an injury and they've been given medication, they become addicted without knowing," said Carolyn Sinclair. "I would say 99% of them said, 'Well, they just told me to take these pills. They'd make me better. I didn't ask if I was going to get addicted to it.' Then they want to go back to work or they're told, 'Okay. You're all better now.' Well, in that line of work, there's certain medications you can't take and be at work. So you stop cold turkey. Now you have no more medication.

"You still may have problems, but you want to get back to work and you're struggling, because you're dealing with the addiction that you may not even have identified as such yet," Sinclair continued. "You can't go back to the doctor and get the medicine. So, they buy it in the places they work. Now they're getting other types of drugs. For some of them it's a huge problem."

What Sinclair was describing was shocking and tragic at the same time. Some of the very same professionals who are responding to illicit drug overdose calls are themselves using those street drugs. This crisis really does have no boundaries.

Heartbreakingly, many people who die from an illicit drug overdose were using secretly and died while a family member, friend, or roommate was at home, perhaps as close as the next room. But because those people had no idea the person was using illicit drugs, or thought they'd stopped using, they didn't know help was needed—until it was too late. Even people who experiment or are occasional drug users are at risk.

———

There's no better time to get married in the Okanagan than late September. After all, this region in the BC Interior, home to world-class wineries and organic orchards, is too scorching hot in the summer to wear a tuxedo. The crystal-clear waters of Lake Okanagan tempt you to jump in just to cool off.

On September 26, 2016, 27-year-old Edmond Paul Adkin was attending a wedding at a hotel in Kelowna—a city on Lake Okanagan just north of towns with such blissful names as Summerland and Peachland. Adkin was an active guy who played lacrosse and hockey as a kid and then rugby in high school, and had recently started playing golf. He'd worked in construction for several years and had just started working for an investment management firm. He had a girlfriend, Talyn.

At 11 o'clock the evening of the wedding reception, members of the wedding party and one of his family members found Adkin unresponsive in a hotel room. He wasn't alone: four other people were in the same room in various states of unconsciousness. An off-duty nurse who happened to be at the wedding quickly came and started CPR on Adkin. Paramedics arrived a few minutes later; they gave naloxone to the five people in distress before taking them to Kelowna General Hospital.

Adkin was in cardiac arrest and having seizures. He was taken to the Intensive Care Unit, but never regained consciousness. He died at 3:00 a.m. on September 28.

"A friend reported that Mr. Adkin purchased what he thought was cocaine from a dealer who delivered it to the hotel," wrote Jacqueline Couch, the coroner who investigated Adkin's death. "Each of the friends used the drugs from the same delivery." Adkin was an occasional user of cocaine and cannabis. The post-mortem toxicology exam found cocaine, a heavy level of alcohol intoxication, and fentanyl. Ms. Couch determined Adkin's death to be caused by anoxic brain injury (lack of oxygen to the brain) due to cardiac arrest caused by mixed alcohol and drug toxicity (cocaine and fentanyl).

All of Adkin's four friends who overdosed that night survived. Fentanyl poses a particularly significant risk to recreational or occasional illicit drug users, like Adkin, who often don't know that the drugs they've purchased contain illicit fentanyl—a substance that their body hasn't developed any tolerance to process.

"Rarely did you see Paul without a smile, or rather a grin, on his face," shared his family. "He was extremely loyal and had a host of close, close friends who will miss him deeply—but will never forget him."

———

Vancouver's Downtown Community Court is located in the heart of the Downtown Eastside, often called the country's poorest postal code. As I arrived at the courthouse at 7:45 a.m., just across the street someone was sleeping outside in the rain under a makeshift shelter. Old tents, tarps, and cardboard boxes. That's what passes as a home in one of the wealthiest countries on earth.

The innovative court was designed to help the criminal justice system recognize that there are underlying health and social issues, including alcoholism and drug addiction, that contribute to offending. It has social workers, mental health workers, and other professionals on site—but it's still a criminal court.

"I have seen, with my own eyes, people in the back alleys in this neighbourhood drawing water into their syringe from a puddle in the lane and injecting it," said Judge Elisabeth Burgess. Using filthy water to dilute powdered drugs so that they can be injected exposes people to risks of disease and infection.

It was clear to me that Judge Burgess has tried to see the world through the perspective of those she judges. When I met with her in a small boardroom before her morning court session began, I asked about her experience with the opioid crisis and the people who end up in her courtroom facing criminal charges.

"I've got a few regulars here—all of them happen to be First Nations—who witnessed their father murdering their mother as small children," said Judge Burgess. "A couple of them actually were so small that they were left with the body for days before anybody discovered it. And, yeah, they're addicts now."

It was a horrific story that transformed the image in my mind of a chronic adult offender, driven by drug addiction to commit petty crimes, into the image of a frightened young child.

Traumatized. Alone. Terrified.

"It's not just that you're necessarily an addict if you had some horrible tragedy in your life. They've got no support," said Judge Burgess. "They've never been diagnosed. They're severely mentally ill. Never seen a doctor. That happens in this city.

"It's a miracle what some of them have been through, but there's that old cliché, and it strikes me every day: the biggest lottery in life is the family you're born into. It's nothing to your credit. You're not better."

I wanted to know more about what role childhood trauma can have on substance use as an adult, and several experts pointed me to the Adverse Childhood Experience (ACE) questionnaire. It asks just 10 yes/no questions about your childhood, but it can tell you a lot about your risk of experiencing a host of challenges later in life. There are questions about physical, emotional, and sexual abuse as well as neglect, parental divorce or separation, incarceration of a parent, and exposure to domestic violence, substance abuse, and mental illness. Each of the 10 questions to which you answer yes counts as a point. These points add up to your ACE score (which ranges from 0 to 10).

Traumatic events and experiences in childhood can lead to social, emotional, and cognitive impairment, which can in turn lead to high-risk behaviours that increase the risk of health problems and premature death. And these harmful childhood experiences can have cumulative effects. For each ACE point, a person's risk goes up for a range of challenges, including poor academic achievement, poor work performance, mental health issues, certain diseases, suicide attempts, and illicit drug use and substance abuse.

A massive study publis'_____ the journal *Pediatrics* found that people with an ACE score _____ who'd experienced at least half of the childh_____ were seven to ten times more likely to hav_____ lem than someone who had an ACE score _____ represents a two- to fourfold increase in the _____ of illicit drugs.

Many people in our _____ ep pain and unresolved trauma. They need o_____ ondemnation. Yet condemnation is precise_____ illicit drugs are treated. As social outcasts. We insist that t___ "personal responsibility" while we ignore our own moral responsibility to help them. More than anything, they're blamed. Blamed for the "bad decisions" or "poor choices" they've made, with no understanding or empathy for how they came to arrive at that place in their lives. They're even blamed for dying.

"People think, 'If you're gonna do drugs, you're asking for it,'" said Shelda Kastor. "'If you're gonna do drugs, tough on you if something happens,' you know what I mean?"

The image of those young children being left alone with their murdered mother for days is etched in my mind. And it speaks of an even longer-term intergenerational trauma that contributed to such a horrific event.

"Their life hasn't worked well. They've had, typically, some blunt-force trauma early in their life and that blunt-force trauma while they're a kid is physical abuse, sexual abuse, verbal abuse," said Bill

Mollard, president of Union Gospel Mission (UGM). His organization runs a network of hot meal programs, shelters, and substance use programs in and around downtown Vancouver. "The drugs, at that point, aren't about partying. They aren't about having a good time. It's about anaesthesia. They use these drugs to mitigate those emotional stresses they have."

Mollard was making a powerful point that's been lost in the public perception of illicit drug use. Synthetic opioids like fentanyl were created to help people endure immense pain as they lay in bed dying. They were intended to numb and block out pain to make life bearable—and that's how people are using them today in the illicit market, too. In other words, absent a properly functioning mental health system and support services, many are self-medicating the pain in their lives.

"Most of the people that I've dealt with in my career have been street entrenched drug users," said Conor King, staff sergeant with the Victoria Police Department. "Almost all of them will tell you a story of things like abuse as kids, disconnection with parents, poverty, trauma in childhood, trauma in adolescence—whether that's domestic violence, sexual abuse, injury or illness when they were in the workforce as a young man or young woman. Despair."

That's where opioids can come into the picture.

"It's got a reputation as something that feels good to take," said Vancouver Fire Chief Darrell Reid in describing fentanyl. "Our patients call it a 'warm hug.'"

Opioids are powerful painkillers. And, unfortunately, there are many, many people with tremendous pain and trauma in our society. We see them now as grown adults, but when we step back and see them as people with lives that are often full of traumatic and painful experiences, holding on to memories that have been unaddressed, and with untreated mental health challenges, we can start to realize that they need our love and compassion.

"There's always this gaping hole in their history that just was not filled by a supportive network—and when later on in life, whether it was as a teenager or as a young adult, they were looking in some way to deal with their trauma, drugs were the answer," said King.

"The intervention that you need for early childhood experience is proper trauma counselling," explained Linda Lupini. "It's not even just 'Mom and Dad think we should all go to see a family counsellor,' because that's happening. It's really good trauma counselling, and that will help mitigate the high risk you're at for addiction."

———

What are other factors that help us understand why people use illicit drugs?

"We look at early drug use, peer influence, trauma, genetics, psycho-social, and mental health concurrent disorders," said Dr. Ronald Joe. "So we can't say that there's a single causative factor. It really depends on each individual person's resilience to trauma and other influences."

I noticed that something was missing from Dr. Joe's list of what causes people to use illicit opioids. Aren't the substances themselves highly addictive? That's always how I'd heard them talked about: the warning to not try them even once or you'll get hooked.

"The vast majority of individuals who take opioids don't have any problems," said Dr. Joe. "The typical person would go for surgery and take some morphine for pain, acute pain, and then we're finding that they don't need to take it anymore."

I had a flashback to when I was in hospital for almost a week as a McGill grad student. I had excruciating abdominal pain. They ruled out appendicitis, but test after test came back inconclusive. Eventually the pain was so bad that they gave me morphine. To me, it felt like an alien presence in my body. I absolutely hated the feeling. The next day, when the pain was resuming, I refused to take it again. Maybe there was something to what Dr. Joe was saying about opioid addiction being much, much more complex and nuanced than the simplistic view we often hear in the media about opioids being "highly addictive" in a physical sense.

"If you put five people on opioids, one person may have an addiction problem. That's based on medical studies," said Dr. Joe. "Nicotine, for instance, is higher. Opioids are actually at the lower end of the spectrum for substances that are potentially habit forming."

The idea of people becoming addicted to drugs based on trying them once, or that there are "chemical hooks" in these substances which are the primary cause of addiction, is a popular urban legend that has been substantially undermined in recent decades. The reasons behind addiction are complex, and our understanding of it is continuing to evolve.

Dr. Joe is quiet-spoken and unassuming. But his low-key demeanour is deceiving: he's a walking encyclopedia when it comes to substance use disorders. He's seen them firsthand, both as a practising physician and now as the medical director of substance use programs for the Vancouver health authority during the opioid crisis.

"I started practising in the Downtown Eastside in the early nineties," said Dr. Joe. "Back then, of course, it was called opioid dependence. It related to the weakness of one's personality and it was a moral issue, and it was something that many of the people who suffered from the condition had control over. Our understanding of it certainly has changed over time."

I'd been struggling to understand why the response to the opioid crisis had been so muted. Why didn't more people care that thousands were dying, and why weren't governments doing more about it? Dr. Joe had just hinted at one compelling reason. Most people don't care about "addicts" (a hurtful and stigmatizing label) overdosing from illegal drugs. They believe that drug users are to blame for harming themselves by "choosing" to use these dangerous illegal substances in the first place: if they overdose and die, it's their own damn fault. It's a harsh form of victim blaming that I started to notice in conversations with even some friends and family members. And it has roots in thoroughly debunked but persistent theories about why people use illicit drugs.

"The Canadian Society of Addiction, the American Society of Addiction, and the [BC] Ministry of Health have all proclaimed opioid use disorder and other addictions as a chronic disease," said Dr. Joe. "That's the best model we have. [And yet] addiction is more stigmatized than the other chronic conditions. We have people who are still of the old mindset and don't really understand the nature of addiction as we currently understand it." Opioid use disorder—characterized by a compulsive and prolonged pattern of problematic use of opioids—is classified as a mental disorder by the American Psychiatric Association in its authoritative *Diagnostic and Statistical Manual of Mental Disorders* (DSM-5, published in 2013).

"There's this whole moral construct around drug use—that the person must be lazy or the person must be weak," said Leslie McBain. "'Why can't they just pull up their socks and get over it and stop?' All of these myths around drug use. We're hoping this is changing. I think it is: slowly in Canada, in BC. Not other places, unfortunately—not south of the border."

"I think we're past thinking that addiction is a moral failure," Bill Mollard told me. "I think we're well past that. I hope we are, because addiction is a medical issue. It is a physiological issue, but it's not solved just by that." Mollard emphasized that many people with substance use disorders are suffering. They need care and compassion, not blame and judgment.

———

Why can't people who are addicted just stop using illicit opioids?

"I think we have to recognize that problematic substance use is a chronic relapsing condition," said Dr. Aamir Bharmal. "To suddenly say that you're just going to be able to get them out and then you've solved the problem—[that] just doesn't happen."

Opioid use disorder is considered to be a compulsive mental disorder. It can start at any age, but it commonly first arises in the late teens and early twenties. It can last for years, even a lifetime. That's because, once people are addicted to illicit opioids, they've lost the ability to simply stop using. They're essentially on autopilot. Their condition is characterized by a strong desire to stop or cut back but an inability to do so. The disorder causes people to take more opioids over a longer time than they intended. Attempts to briefly abstain are typically and quickly followed by relapses.

The condition causes people to use opioids even when it's hazardous to their health and even though they know they're bad for them—which goes a long way towards explaining why so many people are continuing to use street drugs when they know they're likely to be contaminated with fentanyl and fentanyl analogues.

Over time, people with opioid use disorder develop a tolerance to these drugs. That means they need increasingly more to feel the same way. They need greater quantities of the drugs, or more potent opioids. For some long-term daily illicit opioid users, they may actually want fentanyl. "People seek out fentanyl because that's what they know, for one, and then you have a tolerance that develops to a drug that's more potent," said Jordan Westfall. "Basically, when you get used to that, you're going to seek it out because the other stuff isn't going to work for you."

The flip side to developing a tolerance is that if users cut back or stop using for a time, either because they try to abstain or are forced to (e.g., due to being incarcerated), they'll go into withdrawal and their tolerance will reduce rapidly. And when they almost inevitably relapse, their reduced tolerance makes them significantly more likely to overdose. For that reason, abstinence on its own is not recommended as a form of treatment for someone with opioid use disorder.

"If you're an opioid-addicted individual and you're trying very hard to go to recovery, you're at high risk of actually dying," said Dr. Joe. "It's a really cruel chronic disease."

The life of someone with opioid use disorder can be debilitating, and includes being unable to meet major responsibilities at work, school, or home; spending an inordinate amount of time seeking, using, and recovering from using opioids; causing serious problems in relationships with friends and family; and giving up or reducing social, work, and recreational activities.

———

"The kid wanted to get out of this," Leslie McBain told me. Her son, Jordan Miller, had used illicit drugs and was addicted to a mix of prescription opioids. He was trying desperately to stop. "That period between detox and relapse, his girlfriend and I just stuck with him. He had nausea, he had diarrhea, he was trying so hard just to get through it. He had restless arms and legs where his limbs would just fling out. I said, 'Can't you just hold it in?' and he's like, 'No, you can't imagine what it feels like.' You need to do that to release the tension. There's sleeplessness, horrible mood swings. It's nasty."

As McBain put it, "I can imagine people going through withdrawal just giving up and thinking, 'Give me what I need.' Get me that heroin, that fentanyl, that whatever it is, because I can't do this. If you imagine the sickest you've ever been in your entire life, sometimes we say, 'I just wanna die, this is so terrible.' Well, I think multiply that by 10 and you probably have some idea of what it feels like."

Opioid withdrawal typically occurs after someone who's been using opioids for several weeks or more stops or reduces their use. Withdrawal can also be triggered when naloxone (a drug that can reverse an overdose) is given after someone has used opioids. Opioid withdrawal symptoms can occur within minutes and up to several days. They can "cause clinically significant distress or impairment in social, occupational, or other important areas of functioning," and can include the following, according to the DSM-5:

- Dysphoric mood (e.g., depression, anxiety, irritability, inability to concentrate, fatigue)
- Nausea or vomiting
- Muscle aches
- Lacrimation (flowing tears from the eyes) or rhinorrhea (nasal cavity filled with fluid)
- Pupillary dilation, piloerection (hair on skin standing up), or sweating
- Diarrhea
- Fever
- Insomnia

In extreme cases, withdrawal can cause seizures. For many people with opioid use disorder, withdrawal is part of an "escalating pattern in which an opioid is used to reduce withdrawal symptoms, in turn leading to more withdrawal at a later time."

"Most people, when they're addicted to heroin or fentanyl or whatever, they don't actually get high anymore," said Dr. Bonnie Henry. "It's all about trying to stave off those feelings of being dope sick. The withdrawal from it is quite horrendous, makes you feel really bad. So you need more and more just to feel normal again. Opioids change your brain and it resets your normal level, if you will."

Dr. Hasselback has seen the same thing with his patients: "I try to emphasize that there aren't that many users out there that are taking the opioid fentanyl to get high. They're taking it to prevent the withdrawal symptoms. It's the avoidance of the dope sickness that is the major driver to individuals who continue to use illicit drugs."

What exactly is "dope sickness," or withdrawal? How bad is it?

"I mean it's the worst flu, times 100," said Troy Balderson, downtown projects manager at Lookout Society in Vancouver. "It really is that bad. Debilitating. People can't think straight. All you want to do is get well. As you get through it, you get into day three or four, you get hallucinations. I mean it's terrible."

Illicit opioids promise relief from trauma and suffering, often for people who have lost all hope and have nowhere else to turn. They might start as a short-term fix to make the pain go away. And it works, at least for a little while. But then they demand their due, and exact a heavy price. The unresolved trauma and suffering were always there, but now they come back. Added to that are the crippling effects of withdrawal that demand to be satiated—and they won't take no for an answer.

By the time you realize it, it's too late. It's a vicious cycle that exposes that initial promise of a quick relief from suffering as a lie. A cruel hoax that can have deadly consequences.

———

People who regularly use drugs because they're addicted describe the daily struggle they face just to feel some sense of normalcy. Jordan Westfall was one of them. As a university student with a secret, he'd managed to keep up with his studies but was struggling with an increasingly serious substance use problem.

"I was kind of living a double life," said Westfall. "I was a daily opioid user for about five years of my life in my late teens, early twenties. I tried to keep my grades up and at the same time I was dealing with this, which is chaotic. It's exhausting."

Westfall would spend hours every day trying to get access to illicit drugs while juggling a full course load. On days when he wasn't successful he'd go to class feeling like a wreck owing to the harsh and unrelenting symptoms of opioid withdrawal. And on days when he didn't have any money, he'd even sell his textbooks for cash to buy drugs.

OxyContin was supposed to be a temporary fix. But when regulatory changes made these pills much more expensive and, eventually, unavailable on the street, Westfall turned to heroin. "It's almost like if you took food, or took a muffin, and made it illegal and that's your breakfast for the day, but now it's $40 and you have to go hustle on the streets for it. The outcome would be entirely different for a lot of people just to get their breakfast. For us, it puts our lives into chaos." And, of course, your morning muffin isn't laced with illicit fentanyl that could kill you.

Fortunately, Westfall stopped using drugs around the time when he completed his undergraduate degree, just before illicit fentanyl became widespread. He went on to graduate from Simon Fraser University and connected with a group called the Canadian Association of People Who Use Drugs (CAPUD). He says he found acceptance and a platform to call for reforming Canada's drug laws and policies.

By the time I met with him next to the outdoor skating rink at Robson Square in downtown Vancouver, Westfall was leading CAPUD and representing thousands of drug users. In his T-shirt and jeans, he reminded me of many of the law students I've taught over the years. He looked a bit tired (I'm sure I did too), but was bright and engaging. How many of my students were, like Westfall, juggling their studies and their struggles with substance use? How many of them were keeping it secret from everyone? How many of them were, or are, using alone?

Although law schools like UBC have done a lot to raise awareness of and help students with various mental health issues and disabilities, I've never heard of any concrete measures to support students with substance use issues. Meanwhile, the heavy workload, stress, and competition of law school and then legal practice contribute to problematic alcohol and substance use as students and young lawyers grasp for something to relieve the pressure. Some studies have found that one in five lawyers experience problematic substance use—and that the vast majority of those challenges started in law school. It can come with big personal and professional costs. I'm grateful to Westfall for opening my eyes to the opioid crisis that could be in my own classroom and quiet neighbourhood.

Westfall is also concerned about people today who are using alone, despite the prevalent warnings describing the risks of doing so. "First of all, give people a reason to get out of their house. We need to engage with people, and I think that can be done on a community level. If we can get those people to come out and just be like, 'We have a safer option for you when you do it,' we have to be pursuing that."

Westfall had brought it all back to the difficult issue that I knew I'd eventually have to confront when I started this investigation: whether Canada should decriminalize illicit drugs and, even more controversially, whether we should make a "safe supply" available to illicit drug users. Given how miserably the status quo had failed to address the opioid crisis, I'd committed to being open to all options. But I wasn't even close to being convinced yet. I still had too many unanswered questions and a lot more to learn before I could consider something that still seemed so radical.

All this made me wonder: if people who are addicted to illicit drugs can't stop taking them and need support, what was the reason for punishing them with criminalization in the first place?

— 4 —

HAS CRIMINALIZING
DRUGS FAILED?

It was a lot less than what white workers got. In the early 1880s, one dollar a day was all that some 15,000 Chinese workers were paid to finish the transcontinental railway that would connect British Columbia to the rest of Canada. Even worse, these labourers were given the most treacherous jobs. It's estimated that, for every mile of track laid through the Rocky Mountains, one worker died. But no sooner was the railway nearing completion than these Chinese labourers were no longer welcome—and both the provincial and federal governments were determined to send them that message through a series of racial exclusion and discrimination laws.

In Victoria, the BC legislature adopted the Chinese Regulation Act, 1884, which, among other oppressive measures, imposed an annual tax on every Chinese person; required employers to provide a list of all Chinese employees on demand; authorized the creation of toll gates for Chinese people; and placed restrictions on dwellings rented or occupied by Chinese people. This racist law also enacted the first legal prohibition on opioids in Canada. Except for medical or surgical purposes, its use was punishable by a fine of up to $100—the equivalent of approximately $2500 today. Banning opium, which was smoked at the time and had a far lower potency than today's illicit drugs, was part of a suite of measures intended to harass and discriminate against the Chinese population who had brought the practice with them. Indeed, the historical record suggests that the case for prohibiting opium in Canada was racism, pure and simple.

As Dr. Neil Boyd, professor of criminology at Simon Fraser University, told me, "Matthew Begbie, chief justice of British Columbia, held a commission in 1885 that established that smoking opium wasn't nearly as dangerous as alcohol. And that the people who used it were more able to work the next day and didn't get into all kinds of fights that they did in saloons and stuff. There was no need to criminalize."

After the Chinese Regulation Act and other anti-Chinese laws were struck down by the courts, the BC legislature adopted a racist motion calling on the federal government to take action "to prevent our Province from being completely overrun by Chinese."

Sir John A. Macdonald, Canada's first prime minister, was a willing ally. On May 4, 1885, he rose in the House of Commons to personally make the case for excluding Chinese people from voting. "Of course we ought to exclude them," said Macdonald, "because if they came in great numbers and settled on the Pacific coast they might control the vote of the whole Province, and they would send Chinese representatives to sit here, who would represent Chinese eccentricities, Chinese immorality, Asiatic principles altogether opposite our wishes; and, in the even balance of the parties, they might enforce those Asiatic principles, those immoralities which he speaks of, the eccentricities which are abhorrent to the Aryan race and Aryan principles, upon this House."

Macdonald went even further, setting out an astonishingly racist vision for this new country based on theories of white supremacy and racial superiority:

If you look around the world you will see that the Aryan races will not wholesomely amalgamate with the Africans or the Asiatics. It is not to be desired that they should come; that we should have a mongrel race; that the Aryan character of the future of British America should be destroyed by a cross or crosses of that kind. Let us encourage all the races which are cognate races, which cross and amalgamate naturally, and we shall see that such an amalgamation will produce, as the result, a race, equal, if not superior, to the two races which mingle.

On September 7, 1907, rabid anti-Chinese sentiment in Vancouver reached a flashpoint with three days of anti-Asian riots. It began with a parade organized by the "Asiatic Exclusion League," starting at City Hall then proceeding to Chinatown. Twelve-foot-wide banners bore slogans that read "Stand for a White Canada" and "We have fought for the Empire and are ready to fight again." The mob smashed windows and storefronts throughout Chinatown and the Japanese quarters, with several reports of violence against people.

Responding to the 1907 Vancouver riots, the federal government sent William Lyon Mackenzie King, who was then deputy minister of labour but would later become a Liberal prime minister, to investigate. Even though it wasn't in his initial mandate, King wrote a 13-page *Report on the Need for the Suppression of the Opium Traffic in Canada*. It's hardly the stuff of any policy justification I've ever seen: it reproduces his correspondence with the Anti-Opium League, mentions a visit to an opium den and his own over-the-counter purchase, discusses how other countries were dealing with the issue, and includes some newspaper clippings. King argued that prohibition should be national policy and promised it would completely stop the use of opium. He appealed to the moral panic that opium use was causing among white people, particularly concerning young white women. He reproduced the following newspaper clipping in his report:

Awful effects of Opium Habit.

In the police court this morning, while Vancouver lay in the beauty and brightness of early sunshine, there emerged into the light, ugly and horrible evidence of the dire influence which the opium traffic is exercising among the ranks of British Columbia womanhood. May Edwards, pretty and young, had been found in a Chinese den. She said she had a husband in Victoria, and if allowed to go would return to him. She was allowed to go.

Much the sadder of the cases, however, was that of Belle Walker. A terrible record of the effects of indulgence in opium was written upon her appearance this morning. She was found by the police in an opium den. She had been there for three weeks. Magistrate Williams sent her to prison for six months.

In short, the case for criminalizing opioids in Canada in the early 1900s didn't rest on concerns for public health and safety, nor was it founded on any scientific or medical evidence. It was politically motivated, based solely on racism and appeals to moral rectitude.

"Smoking opium was not considered to be physically harmful or socially degenerate," writes Robert Solomon, a professor with the University of Western Ontario Faculty of Law who has researched the history of drug prohibition in Canada. "Yet, the public strongly disapproved of opium smoking among whites, because it involved mixing of the races—a matter considered far more serious than the drug's effects. . . .

"This crusade succeeded because it was directed against Chinese opium smokers and Chinese opium factories, but at the same time posed no threat to the larger number of predominantly middle-class and middle-aged Caucasian users who were addicted to the products of the established pharmaceutical industry."

At the turn of the twentieth century, morphine, heroin, and cocaine were unregulated; they were even found in such products as teething medicine for children, toothpaste, and cough syrup. In fact, as Dr. Scott MacDonald from the Crosstown Clinic pointed out, the word "heroin" was the marketing name given by pharmaceutical company Bayer for its "heroic cough suppressant" that contained the narcotic at the time.

King's report was the launching pad for a national policy of drug prohibition that would criminalize illicit drugs across Canada, with increasingly severe sentences for both users and traffickers. The promise was to eliminate illicit opioid use. More than 110 years later, that promise remains a failure.

———

Despite over a century of trying to eradicate illicit drugs, today the global illicit drug trade is estimated to be worth somewhere between US$426 billion and US$652 billion annually. One of the main goals of the war on drugs—that is, the prohibitionist model—is to eradicate the supply of illegal drugs, or at least disrupt the supply to a major degree, in order to curb drug use and associated criminality. It has failed to achieve that aim.

"The message has to be loud and clear," said Dr. Mark Tyndall, executive director of the BC Centre for Disease Control. "This is a totally demand-driven epidemic." He had a good point, but I wasn't totally convinced until I met his colleague, Dr. Evan Wood, who leads the BC Centre on Substance Use.

Dr. Wood, together with other experts from Canada and the United States, has conducted extensive research into the impact of efforts to reduce the supply of illegal drugs over the last several decades. They used data from the United States, Europe, and Australia, including the inflation-adjusted price of illicit drugs and their average purity (relative potency or strength). The researchers found that not only has it been impossible to address illicit trafficking from the supply side, but that attempting to do so entails serious unforeseen consequences, casting doubt on the whole concept of prohibition.

Between 1990 and 2007, seizures of heroin, cocaine, and cannabis in major production regions and major domestic markets generally increased. The war on drugs was doing what it was supposed to do: cracking down on the supply of illicit drugs in both source and destination countries. What were the outcomes of this apparent success?

Paradoxically, despite massive and incredibly costly efforts to shut down or disrupt their supply, these drugs became cheaper to buy. From 1990 to 2007, the average price of heroin in the United States actually decreased by 81%, the price of cocaine dropped by 80%, and the price of cannabis went down by 86%. Downward price trends were also observed in Europe and Australia.

Even more interesting, between 1990 and 2007 in the U.S., the average purity of heroin increased by 60%, cocaine's by 11%, and cannabis's by 161%. How could that be?

You could call it the law of unintended consequences—by trying to eradicate the supply of these drugs, things were actually made worse as these drugs became less expensive and more potent. That policy outcome is precisely the opposite of what the war on drugs was supposed to accomplish. As drug enforcement intensified and more illicit drugs were seized, illicit drug manufacturers responded by making their products more potent so that they'd be more compact. That way, they could be shipped in smaller quantities that were less likely to be interdicted. Goodbye shipping containers of cocaine from Colombia; hello greeting cards of fentanyl from China.

The war on drugs has also seen unprecedented levels of violence, with global drug cartels, organized crime, and gangs vying for their piece of the pie and battling with police. In many instances, the blood spilled to reap these illicit drug profits has come to the streets, including in major Canadian cities like Vancouver, where innocent lives have been lost in the crossfire.

This whole phenomenon isn't new; it's part and parcel of prohibiting substances. We've seen it before. From 1920 to 1933—the Prohibition era in the United States—there were massive efforts by law enforcement and border agents to shut down the importation and domestic manufacturing of alcohol. That created a huge opportunity for organized crime to make monopoly profits to meet the demand for alcohol products, and led to a lot of bloodshed in the criminal underworld for battles over turf.

Also, since low-alcohol-content products like beer took up a lot of space, they were harder to smuggle. Enter moonshine. Producing spirits with very high alcohol content made the product more compact, so it was harder for law enforcement to detect. But some of these higher-potency products ended up causing blindness and even death. Studies show that, during the Prohibition period, the potency of alcohol products increased by 150%.

In 1986, Richard Cowan, a Republican-turned-cannabis-activist, described this phenomenon as the "Iron Law of Prohibition": "the more intense the law enforcement, the more potent the drugs become." Remarkably, Cowan predicted that potent synthetic drugs would come to dominate the illicit drug market under prohibition, increasing the risk of fatal overdoses. That's right: the current opioid crisis was predicted three decades before it hit a boiling point.

Under prohibition, both suppliers and drug users have strong incentives to minimize the bulk of contraband in order to minimize the risk of detection, thereby encouraging more potent substances.

Sure enough, that's exactly what Dr. Wood and his team's study found to be the effect of trying to shut down heroin, cocaine, and cannabis up to the year 2007. What happened after that date?

The United States dramatically increased its efforts to stop the importation of heroin. Between 2008 and 2015, enforcement at the border with Mexico intensified such that authorities seized 400% more heroin, a staggering scale-up. It was during this same period that OxyContin was transformed into OxyNeo to make it harder to use intravenously. In other words, there were major endeavours to reduce the supply of both licit and illicit drugs.

That's when Cowan's Iron Law of Prohibition kicked in. The criminal underworld found a solution to the crackdown: it started manufacturing illicit fentanyl at a fraction of the price, produced anywhere, and was 30–50 times more potent than heroin. And if that wasn't enough, we're now seeing carfentanyl hitting the streets. It's the Iron Law of Prohibition on steroids.

When I came face to face with the hard evidence, it was clear: the "war on drugs" has not only failed, it's actually made things worse. In fact, it's one of the principal causes of the opioid crisis that has killed hundreds of thousands of people across North America in recent years. In retrospect, the crisis was an entirely predictable consequence of prohibition.

"You know," said Jordan Westfall, "we can play this game for a century. We've already done it, right? I think this has to literally be the death knell of how we do things currently. Like the war on drugs, drug prohibition. If there's a signal in your society that things need to change, it better be 4000 people dying this year of an entirely preventable death. And we're going to continue to lose people at alarming rates unless we do an entire reassessment of how we make policy in this area and how we view people who use drugs."

— 5 —

WHY ARE DEALERS KILLING
THEIR CUSTOMERS?

- *Stir for 15 minutes at 50 to 60 degrees Celsius.*
- *Let cool.*
- *Filter off the salts.*

Five minutes online is all it took for me to find a bona fide recipe for making homemade fentanyl. The underground chemist who published this notorious set of instructions (redacted above) goes by the pseudonym Siegfried. The method was first described in the 1980s—decades before we were introduced to the idea of chemists moonlighting as illegal drug manufacturers like Walter White (a.k.a. Heisenberg) in the HBO series *Breaking Bad*.

"I'm french speaking organic chemist so excuse my rusty english," writes Siegfried. "The risk of overdose is really high, even with the dilution i [*sic*] described before, so test your stuff before selling it!" That advice reminded me of celebrity chef Gordon Ramsay telling aspiring master chefs to always taste the food they plan to serve. Of course, the big difference is that on his show the consequences of making a bad batch are embarrassing, not fatal.

The United Nations Office on Drugs and Crime's 2017 report on fentanyl found that most fentanyl recently seized in the United States isn't pharmaceutical but rather synthesized using Siegfried's method, which doesn't require advanced laboratory skills.

The Siegfried method is just one of several homegrown fentanyl recipes available online that have been verified by Dr. Brian Mayer's team at the Lawrence Livermore National Laboratory in Livermore, California. The 2700 scientists and engineers at this massive national security lab (annual funding: US$2 billion) typically work on research related to weapons of mass destruction and terrorism, so the fact that Livermore has launched a study into illicit fentanyl shows how serious the problem has become. Following these online recipes, Dr. Mayer was able to obtain the necessary ingredients to make illicit fentanyl from commercial chemical suppliers. All it takes is someone with undergraduate-level chemistry experience to do the job, and they don't need fancy lab equipment. Even the precursor chemicals used to make fentanyl can be made relatively easily. But there's a big hitch. While pure fentanyl is relatively cheap and easy to make, diluting it to a consistent dose that humans can safely consume requires much greater sophistication.

Given its high potency, a very small quantity of fentanyl is mixed with buffers such as salt or caffeine; then it's made into pills or cut into other street drugs. And it's at this stage—when fentanyl is fashioned into the final product that will hit the streets—where the real danger arises. The mixing process is often anything but scientific, and the smallest variations can lead to an overdose, or a "hot dose," as it's known. Police have even found kitchen blenders used to mix fentanyl. That's hardly the precise titration used in medical environments where the drug is used as a powerful painkiller.

"Even trying to mix it, because of its high level of toxicity, is very, very difficult, if not impossible," said Clayton Pecknold, assistant deputy minister and director of police services for BC. "You're still running a high risk of a hot dose."

"When we first were detecting fentanyl, I was really under the impression it was a bad product launch," said Dr. Mark Tyndall. "That they really messed up with the dosing, and after a few months they'd sort of get that fixed up. I'm still miffed at the fact that people are selling super potent opioid analogues out there.

"The surprise of the persistence of this crisis is that people are still being exposed to these drugs when I think it's a fixable thing, as far as quality assurance goes. Fentanyl doesn't kill people on its own, but it's just how much you're taking."

Maybe there's a chance that illicit drug producers will get better at dosing so that fewer fatal doses occur, but I wouldn't hold my breath. After all, pure white fentanyl powder may get mixed by ridiculously unsophisticated means before sold to end users. Plus, with the demand for potent fentanyl products, there's an economic incentive for producers to keep products strong, even when that runs the risk of killing some people.

In fact, trafficking fentanyl is so profitable that the loss of some customers from overdose deaths has apparently little to no effect on this lucrative black market. It's like a gold rush—the quickest profit to be earned is the name of the game, with no long-term strategy. And street-level dealers may not even know that they're peddling fentanyl-laced products, although that's become less and less likely as illicit fentanyl has saturated the market.

"Selling opioids is a very profitable enterprise for organized crime," said Inspector Bill Spearn, who heads up the Vancouver Police Department's organized crime section. "They can make a lot more money than they could, say, selling traditional drugs, like cocaine and heroin."

"Everything is profit driven in the drug business," said RCMP Assistant Commissioner Dwayne McDonald. "Like any business, they're pushing the product to get the best bang for the buck."

I heard a wide range of fentanyl profitability estimates from different sources, but they all had fentanyl generating exponential returns. The U.S. Drug Enforcement Administration (DEA) reported that 99% pure illicit fentanyl can be bought from China for between US$3300 and US$5000 per kilogram, and that it can generate revenue in the United States of between US$1.28 and $1.92 million.

Investigators with the Vancouver Police Department keep track of the street price of illicit drugs by doing undercover drug buys and using other investigative tactics. They agreed to share their criminal intelligence data so that I could see just how profitable illicit fentanyl is today compared with a traditional drug like heroin.

In Vancouver, the street price of a hit of illicit fentanyl (3.6% to 5% pure) mirrors heroin—both are $10 for a "half point," or 0.05 grams. Indeed, drug users may think they're purchasing heroin, but end up getting fentanyl. Where things get interesting is that traffickers can import one kilogram of illicit fentanyl (at 51% to 73% purity) for as low as $8600, whereas the same quantity of heroin would cost between $68,000 and $72,000 to import. And remember that fentanyl is many times more potent than heroin. In other words, fentanyl is irresistibly more lucrative for mid- and high-level drug traffickers than heroin.

As Inspector Spearn points out, "You can't even compare fentanyl and heroin. That's why we have such a problem right now. You bring in a kilo of something that is 50 times stronger than heroin for a substantially lower amount of money. It will go 50 times further. The profit is just enormous."

RCMP Sergeant Eric Boechler estimated that, for experienced traffickers, one kilogram of illicit fentanyl can be converted into a multi-million-dollar windfall: "If properly cut for street-level distribution, [it] would be able to create 100 kilograms of counterfeit heroin. Heroin in the Vancouver area typically sells for approximately $70,000 per kilogram, making this 100 kilograms worth approximately $7 million."

But, of course, the cost of this get-rich-quick scheme is being felt throughout North America in terms of lives lost and families suffering, as well as by taxpayers who are footing the bill for massive policing, healthcare, and social services expenditures to respond to the opioid crisis.

"There's so much money to be made, and it sucks that a lot of people really don't care about human life," said Troy Balderson, downtown projects manager at Vancouver's Lookout Society. "They only think about the bottom line, and that's a tragedy in itself."

———

Modern technology has made it easier for mid- and high-level fentanyl traffickers to not only profit from this deadly trade but also avoid detection. Illicit fentanyl, the dark web, and cryptocurrencies have come together in a perfect storm to give organized crime, independent drug dealers, and even individual drug users ready access to overseas illicit drug suppliers. The process offers a lower cost and a reduced risk of detection by law enforcement than does acquiring traditional drugs like heroin or cocaine.

To start with, illicit fentanyl is totally unlike other established street drugs like cocaine and heroin, which require traffickers to move large quantities that are harder to transport surreptitiously. In pure powder form, illicit fentanyl is so potent that even extremely small quantities can turn a massive profit, and they're far less likely to be found by border inspectors. Letters with illicit fentanyl weighing just 10 grams (one-third the weight of a typical greeting card) have been seized at the border. Once they've been delivered, an extremely small quantity of pure fentanyl powder is then mixed, or cut, with other drugs or legal substances like salt and caffeine to expand its volume exponentially.

Another major difference with established street drugs like cocaine and heroin is that these are cultivated in specific locations (such as

Colombia and Afghanistan, respectively), whereas fentanyl is synthetic and so can be produced anywhere. Cocaine and heroin production and distribution are also controlled by extremely violent, hardened criminals. As a warning to others, Mexican drug cartels have allegedly used chainsaws and meat cleavers to behead people who have crossed them.

"You don't have to have that intricate network of connections. It's for sale online," said Victoria Police Staff Sergeant Conor King. "Somebody who is just savvy, wandering through the dark web and savvy with using bitcoin or whatever payment they want to use, can order direct. They don't need to have connections with the Mexican drug cartels or Afghan overlords or whatever. They can just order it online. So it's a simple process. You hear of these people who just order it and UPS delivers it to their door."

The dark web is like a secret part of the Internet that's accessible using special software designed to keep users anonymous and undetectable. It's a whole online world with which most of us are probably unfamiliar. Studies have found that drug trafficking over the dark web is on the rise, although there are also illicit transactions that occur through websites not on the dark web.

How do you pay for goods purchased on the dark web? That's where cryptocurrencies like bitcoin come in. These digital currencies rely on encryption technology to secure and verify transactions. They're virtual mediums of exchange that aren't controlled by any government or central bank and that can later be exchanged for hard cash. And like all technological innovations, the dark web and cryptocurrencies can be used for good or ill.

"Going on the Internet, I was very easily able to find places that would source fentanyl for me and ship it to whatever mailbox and name I wanted," said Abbotsford, BC Deputy Chief Mike Serr, who chairs the Canadian Association of Chiefs of Police Drug Advisory Committee. "I know the RCMP have been doing a significant amount of work on the dark web and places like that to try to source fentanyl."

"We've seen the dark web being used to purchase fentanyl, which means anyone with an Internet connection can generally go online and order it," confirmed David Lothian, chief of the Intelligence Section at the Canada Border Services Agency in BC. According to the U.S. Drug Enforcement Agency, some illicit fentanyl manufacturers in China were once offering customers free replacements if their first order was seized by customs agents. Try getting that kind of customer service from the cartel.

The combination of small quantities of pure illicit fentanyl being ordered on the dark web, paid for using cryptocurrencies, and then shipped by mail or courier delivery is a disruptive game changer for transnational drug trafficking. The model also skirts anti–money laundering and banking regulations designed to combat traditional drug trafficking.

In Canada, all transactions over $10,000 made through a traditional bank get automatically reported to FINTRAC (the Financial Transactions and Reports Analysis Centre of Canada), which has a mandate to detect, prevent, and deter money laundering. But if the quantities of illicit fentanyl being seized are between 10 and 20 grams, then the funds transferred wouldn't automatically be flagged to the authorities. Of course, with cryptocurrencies, transactions of any amount aren't caught. That's a concern for Lothian. "The issue of cryptocurrency is outside our mandate, but it seems that it's still largely unregulated," he told me. "There are challenges in determining how cryptocurrency is defined—whether or not it's a commodity, a currency, or a negotiable instrument. But regulations around that may help because it currently provides the ability for an individual to maintain anonymity through transferring funds and could be used to purchase potential illicit materials like opioids and fentanyl."

But Staff Sergeant King notes that it's not always easy to order illicit drugs online. There are scams out there. Websites offer illicit drugs, then demand payment upfront. They'll happily take your digital currency, but then ship nothing. "I think the problem these guys face is that finding the actual bona fide dealer online, which can deliver, after you send the bitcoin, is harder than it looks," said King. "The Better Business Bureau is not going to be assisting them."

Law enforcement and border officials are scrambling to catch up to the new world they find themselves responsible for policing. And they have a lot of catching up to do. Can we just stop illicit fentanyl from coming into the country, or, as some politicians have argued, can we stop it at its source?

– 6 –

CAN WE STOP FENTANYL
AT ITS SOURCE?

It was March 2013. Undercover officers with the Victoria Police Department didn't know it yet, but the opioid crisis was about to hit British Columbia's coastal city like a tsunami. "We'd known that there was something going on," said Staff Sergeant Conor King. "We wanted to start getting a better handle on it—what drugs were out there."

King's team went undercover to do a drug buy from a local dealer. They didn't know it at the time, but data from the BC Coroners Service would later show that this was almost exactly when illicit drug overdose deaths began to skyrocket in the province.

They had the drugs tested, and there it was: fentanyl.

King immediately contacted the RCMP's CLEAR team (Clandestine Laboratory Enforcement and Response). They were already zeroing in on the source of illicit fentanyl that had started cropping up elsewhere in the country.

"The fentanyl was coming in from China," said King.

Police officers, criminal intelligence analysts, and medical experts all kept telling me that the vast majority of illicit fentanyl in Canada was manufactured in China. (There's a good reason why white-powder heroin laced with fentanyl is called "China White.") The U.S. Drug Enforcement Agency was the most commonly cited source for this information; both the RCMP and the Vancouver Police Department officially cite the DEA. Some police officers and a Crown prosecutor were able to point to investigations and prosecutions they'd run that confirmed the China connection. But a few people I spoke to questioned the China connection, saying it was just hearsay. So I wanted to get direct evidence on the source of the illicit fentanyl that was killing so many thousands of people. That meant getting in touch with the people who protect our borders.

It's tough to get the Canada Border Services Agency (CBSA) to talk much about their work, let alone on the record in a lengthy interview. You might say that the agency is more comfortable asking us questions than answering them. I needed to hear from them directly about whether, and how, illicit fentanyl was entering Canada, and what was being done about it.

To my surprise, I got a quick response to my letter asking to speak with someone at the CBSA about the opioid crisis. Yvette-Monique Gray, director of the Enforcement and Intelligence Division for the Pacific Region, offered to meet me at her office. It turns out that Gray has been a longtime voice for greater openness within the CBSA. Internal emails released under the Access to Information Act in 2010 include her reaction to a reporter's complaint that the agency took three weeks to respond to basic questions about the arrival of a boat of Tamil migrants off the BC coast. She wrote to a colleague, "I know that you'd be preaching to the converted, but it's a vindication of sorts to actually hear a member of the media echo what we think every day. We need to help [the media] by providing the right commentary to them at the right time." It seemed I'd found the right person.

The CBSA office in Vancouver is located in a new glass and metal condominium-style building near the site of the 2010 Olympic Village.

It's an area that used to be rundown, but like much of the city, it has since been gentrified. Now this trendy urban oasis has craft breweries, artisanal ice cream, and access to the seawall boardwalk—far from what you might expect for a government bureau. It's also a stone's throw away from the Downtown Eastside, the part of the city that's been notoriously ravaged by the overdose crisis.

Gray has had an impressive CBSA career, and she often speaks for the agency after major drug trafficking busts. I hadn't been waiting long in the empty CBSA meeting room when Gray entered with David Lothian, chief of the Intelligence Section, who reports to her. After thanking them for agreeing to meet with me, we got down to business.

"For this particular part of the world, because we're so close to Asia Pacific, we put special emphasis on synthetic opioids, on precursors, and definitely on anything that would be coming from Asia Pacific," Gray began.

"We have a large marine port. We have international airports. We have air cargo and we also have an international mail centre as well as a busy land border. But in terms of trade with Asia Pacific, it's significant, particularly the marine port because it's the largest in Canada—and our mail centre also has the most volume from Asia Pacific and from China, which is, of course, where a lot of the opioids come from."

Now I had a basic confirmation of the China connection. But I needed a lot more details. How were illicit opioids entering Canada? What was being done about it? And why can't we just stop illicit fentanyl from entering the country—wouldn't that solve the problem?

"On the mail centre side, we have the biggest mail centre in terms of volume from Asia Pacific and that's where the majority of the fentanyl is that we're seeing, by a long shot," said Gray. "Then also through the air cargo operation, again because of flights from Asia. We have seen quite a bit in the air cargo stream, but for the most part, most of our seizures have been at the mail centre and in the mail stream."

All foreign letters or small packages sent to Canada are routed through one of three international mail centres: Vancouver, Toronto, or Montreal. Most of the international mail going through Vancouver comes from Asia, and it can be subject to the search and seizure of any illegal substances. I knew that Gray couldn't reveal exactly how the CBSA goes about figuring out which letters and packages might contain illicit fentanyl, but I wanted to get a sense of how big a challenge the border agency was facing.

"What's the volume of mail coming through?" I asked.

"On average, the Vancouver International Mail Centre clears about 1.9 million pieces of mail per month from China," said Gray. "That would be everything from letter mail all the way to packages. So generally, the letter mail, it's a flat piece of paper. Obviously you could still put a small amount of fentanyl in there—it would still be worth quite a bit of money and would still be very dangerous—but usually we're seeing it in bigger packages. We're seeing it concealed inside something else. But if you can imagine being able to examine all those individual pieces of letter mail as well as all the larger packages when you're seeing millions in a given month—it would just be impossible."

In that moment, it hit me. There was absolutely no way for us to simply stop illicit fentanyl from entering Canada from China. How could we possibly screen even a fraction of the tens of millions of letters and packages entering Canada every year at this one location? Trying to find illicit fentanyl in that many items would be like looking for a needle in a haystack. And any one of them—even a single letter—could contain enough fentanyl to be worth thousands of dollars and to kill hundreds of people.

"We do have the obligation to facilitate the free flow of legitimate trade and to make sure that goods continue to move," added Lothian.

Indeed, massive quantities of legitimate "Made in China" goods are imported into North America, making it easier for fentanyl to enter undetected. "Obviously we couldn't shut down the mail centre entirely just to strictly look for fentanyl. There's such a major economic and financial implication to doing something like that."

Remarkably, it wasn't until May 18, 2017—several years into the opioid crisis—that the CBSA finally got the legal authority under the Customs Act to open incoming international mail weighing 30 grams (the weight of a typical greeting card) or less. Before that, they couldn't even touch most letter mail. Still, with CBSA's mail seizures typically measuring between 10 and 200 grams of pure fentanyl, traffickers can reduce the risk of detection by spreading it in small quantities across dozens or hundreds of packages (although frequent packages to the same address could get flagged).

Risk management is also the way the CBSA prioritizes its work. Identifying which letters and packages to check is an exercise in focusing your resources on what analysts estimate to be the greatest probability of the worst harm.

"We do have X-rays," said Gray, seemingly trying to restore some confidence in the screening process that, from where I sat, would never be adequate to the challenge she'd described. "If something is concealed inside something else, you can see it through an X-ray. Is it heroin? Is it fentanyl? Is it cocaine? You don't know what it is, but you know there's something that doesn't belong there. So all of the high-risk mail is actually examined either by X-ray or it's examined manually by opening it. But the other part that's been different for us, and it was a game changer, is the health and safety issues associated with handling fentanyl."

Not only is it impossible for border agents to check all envelopes and packages for illicit substances, but opening one that's suspected of containing fentanyl is a complicated process. The CBSA got some advice from the RCMP's CLEAR team about how to do it. "Our officers need to open packages with extra caution, including using things like fume hoods, to ensure there is no contamination," said Gray. "If it's steroids and you open it and white powder goes in the air, you're not as concerned. If it's fentanyl, you're concerned." While I could imagine the need for caution in opening these packages, in other contexts, several of my sources noted that claims of people overdosing just from touching fentanyl are the stuff of urban legend that simply increase the stigma against people who use drugs.

Even if a suspicious substance is uncovered, there's no way of knowing what it actually is until it's been tested. Those tests used to be done by the CBSA's central drug lab in Ottawa, but the opioid crisis changed all that. The process was just too slow. "We have had a satellite lab actually set up where they were able to test substances immediately," said Gray. "So it gave the officers a greater level of comfort with examining it, and the feedback on what is and isn't fentanyl is a lot faster because the lab was right there."

With the massive volume of letters and courier packages coming through the Vancouver International Mail Centre, it's amazing that any pieces containing the deadly substance are found at all. When I asked Gray about how successful the agency has been at interdicting illicit fentanyl, she promised to get back to me with concrete statistics. Just a few weeks after we met, she emailed me the numbers.

In 2017, the CBSA made 47 illicit fentanyl seizures (weighing a total of 7.5 kilograms) from letters and packages at the Vancouver International Mail Centre. An additional six packages were seized that were being sent via courier companies with illicit fentanyl weighing a total of 2.2 kilograms. So, in all, less than 10 kilograms of illicit fentanyl was seized from 53 items in 2017—about one seizure per week on average. This illicit fentanyl, in pure form, was prevented from hitting the streets. But if we're honest, we know that it's just a drop in the bucket. That's 53 items identified from around 22.8 million in one year: 0.0002% of total packages. We're never going to be able to solve this problem at the border.

———

What about at the source? If we can't stop illicit fentanyl from entering Canada at our borders, what about getting China to crack down on this deadly export at its end? After all, it's being produced within their territory; they should be responsible for the harm it's causing.

A big part of the challenge is that, unlike many other illicit narcotics, fentanyl has legitimate medical purposes. There are thousands of legal pharmaceutical labs in China, and it's not clear to what extent illicit fentanyl products coming from China to North America are being diverted from these legal labs, illegal labs, or both. "In trying to determine where illicit drugs are being made, and given the fact that there is a legitimate market for fentanyl, we try to determine if it could possibly be diverted from a legitimate factory for illicit purposes," said Gray. Abbotsford, BC Deputy Chief Mike Serr echoed Gray's concern: "Many of them are producing it actually legally, but then also have a subset of their company that is also shipping this out illicitly as well."

Another key player in responding to the opioid crisis on Canada's West Coast is Clayton Pecknold. He served as co-chair of BC's overdose task force that was set up to deal with the opioid crisis, and is an assistant deputy minister and director of police services for BC. "There was a period of time where we were advocating for an agreement with China to interdict fentanyl from China," he told me. "We, the province of BC, had raised that with the federal government. It was not in place, notwithstanding that the federal drug agency in the United States, the DEA, had already entered into one with China. It's not that the RCMP don't know how to do their job. They know how to do their job. Unfortunately, they were underfunded federally for so long and they were so focused on counter-terrorism that they haven't had the capacity to do the type of early warning intelligence gathering that they should be doing on the drug file."

On November 24, 2016, the RCMP and the Chinese Ministry of Public Safety announced that they would coordinate enforcement against illicit fentanyl trafficking. China also agreed to make precursors (substances that can be used to make fentanyl) controlled under Chinese law. This has meant that some limited progress has been made. "Hong Kong Customs does do outbound checks, and has intercepted fentanyl previously," Gray told me. "When they intercept something like fentanyl, they will often alert us to the fact that they've made a seizure on export. Those outbound seizures have provided us with valuable intelligence information, and have assisted us with our efforts to identify drug smuggling groups within Canada."

Yet, while the level of cooperation from Chinese authorities at their end of the transnational drug trafficking chain isn't insignificant, there's a heavy dose of pessimism to counter whatever optimism exists for China's ability to shut off the export of illicit fentanyl. And part of that lies in the drug's chemical makeup.

———

Fentanyl ($C_{22}H_{28}N_2O$) is actually fairly straightforward, comprising four basic elements: carbon, hydrogen, nitrogen, and oxygen. By making a few changes to its chemical structure, an "analogue" can be created. Think of an analogue as a copy, but with very minor changes. It's alike enough to provide similar or enhanced effects, but just different enough that at the molecular level it's technically another substance.

The most infamous fentanyl analogue is carfentanyl ($C_{24}H_{30}N_2O_3$), although there are in fact dozens of them, many of which have no medical use. Some have been rediscovered by illicit drug manufacturers from research carried out since the 1960s, while others are new "designer drugs" created by chemists working for the benefit of organized crime. Why all the variations on fentanyl? To keep one step ahead of the law.

Drug regulation in many countries, including China, is based on "scheduling" specific substances—identifying them by their chemical composition. These scheduled drugs are then subject to strict controls, meaning they can be legally manufactured only in certain facilities and sold only for certain purposes. And as more fentanyl analogues get scheduled, chemists working at the behest of organized crime have that much more incentive to come up with new ones. "Once an announcement is made about regulating new substances or analogues," Lothian told me, "then it's usually within a month or two months that we start to see new analogues that we hadn't seen previously that do try to bypass some of those regulations."

For years, when new fentanyl analogues were detected in Canada and the United States, authorities here would complain to China, which would then add them to their list of scheduled substances, meaning they fall under legal regulation. Then, within a month or two, a new fentanyl analogue would be discovered on the streets here; it would get reported and then added to the schedule in China, and on it went. Given the massive profits involved and the ingenuity of these chemists of death, this deadly game continued. It was not until May 1, 2019 that China finally adopted a class-wide control of all fentanyl-like substances.

Rapidly evolving analogues can also make it tougher to detect and identify new substances as a form of fentanyl. "The way detection technology works around this, sometimes you tweak two things and all of a sudden your detection technology that was working really well doesn't indicate to the same level," said Gray. "So that analytical piece is really critical to staying ahead of all of these compounds."

Despite reportedly seizing 1.8 tonnes of illicit drugs between 2015 and 2017, China shut down only eight production labs—and this in a country with an estimated population of 1.4 billion. Still, China is the first to admit that it can't get ahead of the illicit drug manufacturers exporting their deadly products to the world. "My feeling is that it's just like a race and I will never catch up with the criminals," said Yu Haibin, a division director at the Chinese Ministry of Public Security's Narcotics Control Bureau. The likelihood of China being able to stop the outflow of illicit fentanyl analogues seems remote.

But what if China *does* become really good at cracking down on illicit fentanyl manufacturing and transnational trafficking? Criminal opportunists are undoubtedly waiting in the wings to pick up any slack. There are already indications that other global players in the drug trade, particularly Mexico, are involved in making illicit fentanyl. According to the U.S. DEA, "Both Mexico and China are major source countries for fentanyl and fentanyl-related compounds" (although drug seizures in the United States have found that fentanyl from China is generally higher in purity than that from Mexico). Still, as Lothian told me, "We have heard of intelligence reports about Mexico producing fentanyl, but we actually haven't seen a lot of fentanyl come through our land borders or come through that network." In central and eastern Canada, the CBSA has also found fentanyl entering Canada by mail from various European countries in the form of pills and fentanyl patches.

In short, if China manages to turn off the tap, there are dozens of countries with lax regulations, corrupt officials, and organized criminals that would jump at the opportunity to take over its role as the world's main illicit fentanyl supplier. It's the globe's deadliest game of whack-a-mole waiting to be played: every time one supplier gets hit, another one pops up to take its place.

———

So far, we've seen that most illicit fentanyl entering Canada is coming from China, hidden among the millions of items every month entering Vancouver by post. The dark web and cryptocurrencies are being used to conceal the identities of purchaser and seller, skirting anti–money laundering and banking rules that have been developed over decades to combat transnational drug trafficking. But what about the relatively small number of letters and packages entering the country that, despite the astronomical odds, *are* intercepted by border agents? If they've got a package made out to a Canadian address and containing pure illicit fentanyl, surely they could nab the person who ordered it in Canada, right? That's what I wanted to know from Gray and Lothian at the CBSA.

"You've opened a package. You've inspected it. You've got white powder. It then tests positive for fentanyl. What happens next?" I asked.

"Once we have confirmation that it is a controlled substance, we will continue working with whatever information is available," said Lothian. "We look into the importer name and address, the exporter name and address, and look for any linkages or commonalities to previous seizures. A lot of that data is, at times, fictitious, because you can write whatever you want onto a package. So it's definitely challenging to make some linkages to who is ultimately behind some of these shipments." But the CBSA doesn't operate alone. "We'll work with our police partners and we'll refer the file to them," Lothian continued. "Collectively we'll work out an investigative approach to try and see if we can determine who is responsible for that importation and proceed that way."

That sounded promising, but something didn't make sense. Why had none of the police officers I'd interviewed told me about charging Canadian-based buyers with importing illicit fentanyl based on being tipped off by border agents? That would be a major charge, warranting some serious jail time. When I asked for more details Gray stepped in, drawing on her years of experience as a customs officer and now director.

"If someone has cocaine strapped to their body and they come through the airport and say they didn't know how that cocaine got there, no one believes that," she said. "If someone is driving in a vehicle, there might be a little bit more plausible deniability if they say 'This isn't my car.' But if something is sent through the mail and if it contains contraband, when we or our police partners conduct our follow-up investigation they can say that they weren't expecting a letter, it was mistakenly sent to them, or they don't know the person that sent it. So the deniability goes through the roof. One of the biggest problems with anything coming through the mail is, how do investigators prove this person knew that this was being mailed to them? So the standard of proof is so much higher. If it now happens five times, well, it's harder to say that you didn't know. 'Why would they keep using your address?' But if it happens once, it's very easy for them to just say, 'I don't know. I have no idea.'"

These sounded like massive challenges in prosecuting Canadian-based illicit fentanyl importers, but there had to be a way around them. I'd heard somewhere about an investigative technique called a "controlled delivery." Basically, when law enforcement officers detect a package containing illicit drugs in transit, they allow it to go forward under their control and surveillance, then arrest the person who receives it once they've accepted it. With a substance like illicit fentanyl, it could be replaced with a decoy that looks similar. Couldn't that technique be used by police? I decided to ask the Vancouver Police Department's top drug investigator.

"In fact, it's illegal for us to interfere with the mail, and that's where all these opioids are coming into Canada," said Inspector Bill Spearn.

It didn't make sense at first. Can't the police get a warrant from a judge to seize these illegal substances? I'd read my Criminal Code, but not the Canada Post Corporation Act. Inspector Spearn had.

It turns out that under our federal postal legislation, "nothing in the course of post is liable to demand, seizure, detention or retention." The provision appears to be written to override powers that the police have under the Criminal Code. I had no idea. Although the CBSA can seize packages entering Canada, the police aren't allowed to meddle with the mail. Needless to say, this poses a big challenge for them, given that our taxpayer-funded postal system has been co-opted by drug traffickers to ship illicit fentanyl with impunity.

And it's not just fentanyl. According to the RCMP, cocaine, heroin, guns, grenades, stun guns, and even a rocket launcher have also been shipped via Canada Post.

"We need changes in the Canada Post Corporation Act to allow the police to legally intercept the mail, with the proper authorizations, of course," Inspector Spearn told me. And indeed, the Canadian Association of Chiefs of Police has asked the federal government to allow police to obtain an order from a judge to seize, detain, or retain letters or parcels being sent through Canada Post that contain illicit contraband. "They've been trying to change that now for five years," said Spearn. "The Liberal government came out and said that they weren't going to amend that Act. We can't even reinsert a placebo back in the mail to do a controlled delivery, because putting it back in the system is interfering with the mail."

Even if police had that ability to intercept mailed items with a judge's authorization, there's another dilemma. Letters and packages containing illicit fentanyl are often addressed to post office boxes. "They let it sit there for a week or two to ensure that it's not going to be intercepted by the police," said Deputy Chief Serr. The cost of running an undercover police surveillance team for two weeks at a post office—which, in high-risk situations like drug surveillance, could include both a surveillance and a counter-surveillance team— would be hundreds of thousands of dollars. And even if they did secure a prosecution, the quantity involved in such a seizure would be small. Simply put, in a world of scarce policing resources, it wouldn't pass the cost/benefit analysis that drug investigators have to make in deciding where to prioritize their efforts.

The importation of illicit fentanyl—where the chances of being caught are so low and the profits so high—is a Wild West, and everyone involved knows it. The authorities are trying to fight the opioid crisis with their hands tied behind their backs.

——

Is there any indication that fentanyl is being manufactured here in Canada? There's some evidence of these secret labs, but given China's massive supply role, they're currently believed to play an insignificant part. As Pecknold told me, "Well, we keep hearing it. I haven't seen any actual production labs cross my desk, and I get pretty well informed by the RCMP. We have had methamphetamine labs here; we have had other production facilities, but in terms of actually producing fentanyl, carfentanyl, we haven't seen that yet. At least it hasn't been reported to me."

Assistant Commissioner Dwayne McDonald, the officer in charge of the RCMP's Surrey detachment, said: "We get a lot of what I refer to as production. It's usually where we get involved—it's the cutting of it, or the pill pressing of it. They'll be mixing it into either legitimate drugs, or they might mix it with heroin or might mix it with cocaine or mix it with caffeine and aspirin to make a counterfeit OxyContin pill."

At any rate, the RCMP has put out an awareness notice for landlords about potential signs that a tenant may be running an illicit fentanyl lab on their property. They say that "micro-labs" could be in homes and apartments, motels, rental trucks, abandoned buildings, barns, and even garden sheds, and they've listed their warning signs:

- Unusual amounts of white or coloured powder on walls, floors, countertops, furniture, clothes dryer and/or vent
- Unusual thumping sounds that could indicate a pill press machine
- Chemical odours—often a strong vinegar smell
- Tenants reluctant to allow landlords to inspect the property
- Payment of rent in cash
- Surveillance cameras
- Curtains always drawn
- Exhaust fans running at odd times. Residents may wear filtration masks, safety glasses or other protective equipment. May remark that they are "painting."

And if you suspect a fentanyl lab, the RCMP advises that you not investigate or enter the area but rather leave right away and contact them.

There is some circumstantial evidence of potential domestic fentanyl production, according to Deputy Chief Serr. "We're seeing a lot of precursors that are coming in as well, which would be used not only for meth but also for fentanyl."

I wanted to follow up with the Canada Border Services Agency to see what they were finding. Sure enough, "We certainly have seen some chemical precursors that could be used in the manufacture of opioids and fentanyl," Lothian told me. "We also have seen certain lab equipment that gets imported—for example, things like pill presses or chemical mixing machines and things like that." Gray added, "It's really important for us and our law enforcement partners to look at the precursors and make sure we're watching for signs of domestic production to ensure that Canada does not become part of a pipeline." Dr. Richard Frank at Harvard confirmed that raw materials for manufacturing fentanyl and some of the necessary equipment are also entering the United States from China.

But the only concrete reference I found to domestic manufacturing in Canada came from the United Nations Office on Drugs and Crime's 2017 fentanyl report. It identified three cases of varying levels of sophistication: an industrial-scale facility, a medium- to large-scale facility, and a lab in someone's kitchen. Interestingly, each of these was busted in 2011–2012, predating the current opioid crisis. It's also unclear whether these cases involved simply mixing imported fentanyl or actually creating it.

In sum, then, although illicit fentanyl is not believed to be manufactured domestically to any significant degree yet, powdered white fentanyl is being brought into Canada to facilities where it's cut and mixed to make illicit drug products that can be sold here on the street or through "dial-a-dope" home delivery operations.

But if we get better at interdicting fentanyl entering Canada, do we run the risk of seeing more domestic production, sort of like what we've seen with previous synthetic drugs like methamphetamine?

"Yeah," said Pecknold. "That's a concern. For sure. We're on the lookout for that." But, as Deputy Chief Serr told me, "There really isn't a lot of reason to invest in making a lab. I do think that if down the road we're able to stem the flow a little bit we will for sure see more labs. But at this point, I can go on my Internet right now, in my basement, and order it through the dark web and have it delivered to my mailbox with very little risk."

———

I had one last question: Is there a way to identify the specific source of illicit drugs when someone overdoses?

"That's something that I think is hard to track," said Andy Watson with the BC Coroners Service. "But right now, we don't have the mechanism to be able to find out where it's come from."

That's exactly what forensic scientists have been trying to figure out at the California-based Lawrence Livermore National Laboratory.

Since fentanyl is a synthetic drug that can be made in a number of ways, it has what are known as "chemical attribution signatures." These signatures provide details about the final chemical composition of the drug as well as clues to how a given sample was made, what precursors were used, and what its by-products are. Dr. Brian Mayer's team at Livermore has even been able to capture this kind of information from fentanyl residue on surfaces that are typical in the real world, like stainless steel and vinyl tile. It's neat science, but it doesn't claim to be a silver bullet for investigators. It may point them only in a certain direction. And, at the end of the day, it probably doesn't matter anyway.

"I mean, it's just a synthetic product. So this idea that we can shut it off—it's kind of a joke," said Dr. Mark Tyndall. "If we couldn't stop heroin coming in, how the hell would you ever stop fentanyl from coming in in tiny packages and stuff?"

−7−

WHO'S BEEN
HARDEST HIT?

Panoramic ocean views, majestic sunsets, cozy Adirondack chairs surrounding a crackling fire pit, a relaxed, small-town feel. A paradise on earth. It must have seemed the perfect place for Brandon Jansen to start again.

On March 1, 2016, the fit 20-year-old arrived at the Sunshine Coast Health Centre in Powell River, BC, after being released from jail. The private treatment centre is for people with substance use disorders, and couldn't be in a more beautiful part of the world.

Brandon's mother, Michelle, was desperate to help her son with his opioid addiction. He'd been in and out of prison three times already, each time released to a different drug treatment centre. In all, he'd tried 11 detox centres, recovery homes, and treatment centres since 2013.

Michelle had spent over $200,000 on private treatment to help her son. Some of the residential programs had cost between $25,000 and $30,000 a month. For those Canadians who could manage that at all, it could mean remortgaging their home, cashing out their retirement savings, or both. But what else can you do when your child's life is on the line?

"Brandon had a smile that lit up a room and always had a twinkle in his eye," said his family. "He enjoyed hunting and fishing. He dreamed of opening his own fitness centre and supplement store."

But less than a week after checking into Sunshine Coast, Brandon was really starting to struggle again. He told staff he was thinking about drugs and feeling anxious. They gave him extra anti-anxiety medication at 11:45 p.m., but Brandon couldn't get to sleep. He went outside to have a cigarette with two other clients at the centre and returned to his room at 2:45 a.m.

At 5:00 a.m., another client from the centre went into Brandon's room and found him on the floor, his body crouched up. The client called for help. Brandon wasn't breathing and his skin was cold and purple. They called 911, began performing CPR, and used a defibrillator to try to revive him.

Clients at the centre told the paramedics they thought Brandon had overdosed, likely on fentanyl. They gave him a shot of naloxone to try to reverse the effects of the overdose and continued life-saving efforts for another 30 minutes. On the advice of the emergency physician, they finally stopped. Later it turned out that Brandon had died at least 20 to 30 minutes before the paramedics arrived.

A coroner's inquest heard from 35 witnesses. It concluded that the immediate cause of death was an accidental mixed opioid drug overdose. The toxicology report found fentanyl, acetyl fentanyl (a fentanyl analogue), and heroin in his system.

That's not all the coroner's inquest found.

"Brandon was an engaging young man who seemed motivated to attend treatment," said Michael Egilson, the presiding coroner who investigated Brandon's death. "The pathologist concluded that as Brandon had not been using illicit opioid drugs recently, his drug tolerance would have been lowered, resulting in his death."

The combined effect of being incarcerated, where access to illicit opioids is limited, and the abstinence program that Brandon was on meant that his tolerance to opioids was greatly reduced. That put him at greater risk of overdosing when he used again. Remember that opioid use disorder is a chronic, relapsing condition. No matter how badly Brandon wanted to, he couldn't just stop using on his own.

———

Under India's traditional caste system, the lowest of the low, known as the "untouchables," faced social ostracization, segregation, and discrimination. But every society, including Canada's, seems to have its own version—groups of people treated as second-class citizens or worse. An outside observer would reasonably conclude that criminals, Indigenous people, and the poor constitute Canada's untouchables due to how they're treated in our society. Statistics bear this out: these three groups are among the most vulnerable to illicit drug overdose deaths, and during the opioid crisis it is they who've been disproportionately killed.

The 2003 SARS epidemic killed 44 people in Canada and generated a massive mobilization of public resources to contain its spread. Hundreds of times that number have died in this country from opioid-related overdoses in recent years. Why has the response to these deaths not been proportionate?

Simply put, the lives of drug users (especially when they're criminals, Indigenous, or poor) aren't valued by our society. These are socially and politically marginalized groups that elicit little sympathy and attention from governments. And, as we've seen, people with substance use disorders are wrongly blamed for their misfortune.

But we don't have to accept this. Gandhi called the untouchables children of God and worked tirelessly for their social acceptance and inclusion. Jesus led by example by regularly spending time with the social outcasts of his era, healing those with all manner of conditions and appealing to us to love and care for those less fortunate. Martin Luther King, Jr. declared that all are created equal and dreamed of a day when that would become a reality. The Canadian Charter of Rights and Freedoms guarantees the right to equal protection and equal benefit of the law without discrimination. Either we value the lives of others and care for them or we think we're better than they are and ignore their suffering. Whether our reasons are faith-based, grounded in respect for human rights and dignity, or based on life experience, if the opioid crisis is to be given the resources and attention it deserves, we need a groundswell of care and compassion to bubble up across a wide cross-section of society.

I was involved in politics for almost two decades and saw firsthand that when a problem affects a group of people who are politically important (e.g., those who are organized and mobilize, vote in large numbers, donate to political parties, and can garner media attention), their issues get quickly addressed. I've also seen how challenges faced by marginalized and disadvantaged groups who lack that political power tend to be ignored indefinitely. Unless others who can get noticed speak up alongside them, nothing will change. Indeed, that's one of the main reasons I wrote this book. I couldn't stand by as so many people were being senselessly slaughtered by the silent death of opioid overdose.

———

Soon after the inquest into Brandon Jansen's death, the presiding coroner, Michael Egilson, was tasked with leading a comprehensive "death review panel" that would investigate every single illicit drug overdose death in BC between January 1, 2016, and July 31, 2017. The goal was to identify trends to help prevent further loss of life.

It was a painstaking, file-by-file review of all 1854 deaths during that period.

When I read Egilson's report it came as a real shock. During my research interviews only a few experts had even hinted at his major finding, and none of those individuals were professionals in the criminal justice system.

Egilson found that 18% of those who'd had a fatal illicit drug overdose died while under community corrections supervision or within a month of being released from jail. Brandon Jansen was one of them. There's more: a full 66% had been involved with BC Corrections at some point in their lives or were under supervision when they died. It's a surprising statistic that reveals a massive connection between the criminal justice system and fatal overdose deaths. Why?

To start with, Egilson confirmed what researchers had been saying for years, even before the opioid crisis: people released from jail are at high risk of dying from a drug overdose. The first two weeks after release are especially dangerous.

"Their tolerance is lowered," said Linda Lupini with BC Emergency Health Services. "So, now what? So now they go straight to where they buy something on the street, not knowing what's in it. Their tolerance is lower, and they die unless somebody sees them or we get called. So we do see a high proportion of people coming out of correctional facilities."

The same phenomenon has been observed in the United States. "While there is access, obviously, to drugs in prisons, it's not the same as on the street," said Dr. Richard Frank. "People were used to using certain doses when they go into prison. They're not getting that anymore, and then they come out and go back to their old dose—and they basically immediately overdose because their bodies haven't been acclimatized to that anymore."

In his medical practice in the Downtown Eastside, Dr. Ronald Joe, medical director for substance use services at Vancouver Coastal Health, has seen many people with opioid use disorder who've recently been released from jail. He told me about the lengths to which one of his recent patients went to get help after being tossed out of pre-trial custody without any support whatsoever. "He had a few scratches on his face," Dr. Joe told me. "I said, 'How are you feeling? You look a little bit ruffled up,' and he said, 'Yes. I'm a bit ruffled up. I was released from prison and I actually hiked here from Coquitlam to the Downtown Eastside. I know all the special trails. That's why I have some scratches—from a few branches here and there.'"

I asked Dr. Joe why this man had hiked over 30 kilometres to come to his clinic.

"He was released without a prescription," he responded. "So he just came for a prescription."

"For what?"

"Opioid agonist," said Dr. Joe, referring to Suboxone or methadone—medications that would help prevent his client from going into withdrawal, which would have made him more likely to use illicit opioids and overdose.

It's remarkable what people like Brandon Jansen and Dr. Joe's patient will do to seek help for their opioid use disorder. It upset me to hear how the corrections system was leaving them at greater risk of overdosing just when they want to get help. And the risk of a fatal overdose after release from custody actually persists for years. According to Egilson, 44% of those who fatally overdosed and had been in custody died within two years of being released. So much for helping people reintegrate into society and rehabilitate.

People in custody should have equal access to the medical interventions and evidence-based treatment options discussed later in this book. It's in their best interest, and it's in society's best interest. Right now, though, they're basically tossed out with little, if any, support. And like Brandon, each of them is somebody's son or daughter.

———

East Hastings and Main streets intersect at the epicentre of Vancouver's Downtown Eastside, where one of the most visible homeless populations in Canada can be found. Many here suffer from serious untreated mental health issues, fetal alcohol spectrum disorder, physical disabilities and injuries, and substance use disorders. There's also a notable proportion of Indigenous people.

Groups of people mill around while others sit on pieces of cardboard. The long lines are for warm meals offered by local charities. Parts of syringes litter the sidewalks despite efforts to clean them up. There are people in wheelchairs struggling to cross the busy streets in time—one man backs his wheelchair across, kicking the ground with his foot to slowly propel him along. Shopping carts are filled with a person's earthly belongings. A man rocks rhythmically back and forth facing a brick wall. There's the acrid smell of urine near the alleyways. Others lie on the hard concrete, wrapped up in distinctive thin white blankets with blue lines; I recognize these from the hospital.

"Most of us are just a couple of paycheques, one injury on the job, or one mental health crisis away from homelessness," said Jennifer Breakspear, executive director of PHS Community Services Society.

Places like the Downtown Eastside and the tent cities found in many other places are Canadian skid rows. I'm always baffled—and annoyed—when some journalists call these homeless people "campers," as if they're on some sort of pleasant vacation with campfire singalongs and marshmallows.

Despair and drug use are frequent companions. It's not surprising that there are so many overdoses among people who are homeless or living in precarious housing, whether these be emergency shelters, temporary housing, or ultra-low-rent (and often derelict) single room occupancy (SRO) facilities.

"Welfare Wednesday" is a day that first responders in these areas dread. They know that it brings a spike in illicit drug overdose calls, and that more people will die. It's the day when monthly income assistance cheques are given out in BC—cheques that barely cover a rundown room and subsistence expenses. The amount of money for food works out to just $19 a week, less than $1 a meal. Try living on that. I did, as part of the 2017 annual #welfarefoodchallenge organized to raise awareness. I lost several pounds and felt lethargic. I was constantly hungry, unproductive at work, and cranky at home. And that was after just a week. In 2018 the challenge was cancelled because rising costs meant that the amount of money left over for food would be just $6 a week—less than a dollar a day. Living long-term on that pittance would lead to countless health problems and affect you in myriad ways. But even food takes a backseat when you have opioid use disorder. That's how powerful it is.

"When you get money as an addicted substance user, it's your first thought," said Troy Balderson, downtown projects manager with Lookout Society. "It really is. Before food. Before anything, you want to take that pain away, whether it's traumatic pain, whether it's emotional pain, or whether it's physical pain."

As Andy Watson with the BC Coroners Service told me, "On the five days that follow income assistance payments, we're seeing almost double the number of deaths per day than we do on other days of the month. For 2017 alone I believe it was almost six deaths per day . . . whereas in the rest of the month we were closer to three."

"This past Wednesday," said Linda Lupini, "we did 104 overdoses." She explained that, right across the province, there's usually double the number of 911 overdose calls on income assistance Wednesdays (a typical day will see 50 to 60 overdose calls). "Sometimes we start to see people the day before because sometimes they go to Money Mart."

———

Coastal BC's temperate climate is a draw for homeless people from across the country. After all, it's next to impossible to live outdoors in the frigid weather most of the rest of Canada endures during its snowy winters. Another prominent reason the Downtown Eastside always seems to be attracting people is the access to services. The fact that a sizable proportion of Downtown Eastside residents have serious mental health challenges is partly related to the 2012 closure of nearby Coquitlam's Riverview mental health facility, which advocates say occurred without any real plan to help patients afterwards.

"Somewhere between 20 to 30% of the folks who come to access care are newcomers to the Downtown Eastside. It's up each and every year," said Dr. Joe. "They come from adjoining jurisdictions, whether it be proximal—Burnaby, Surrey, and further north, Prince George and so on—or from back east. You have people from Alberta, Saskatchewan, and Ontario. The issue of the Downtown Eastside isn't an issue of the residents of the Downtown Eastside. It's actually a Canadian issue."

At Vancouver's Downtown Community Court, that's been Judge Elisabeth Burgess's experience, too. "This is a place that's been made more supportive, and services are available. You can live here on the street," she pointed out. "It's not something I'm recommending, but it's doable, and of course our climate makes a difference to that as well. There have been estimates of how much money gets poured into the Downtown Eastside on a daily basis, and the lowest I've seen is a million dollars a day for services.

"Every day in court I listen to people talking about how 'I came here from'—naming the other province—'because I thought it would be easier.' But a lot of them say their life's just gone to hell because drugs are so much more easily accessible here—illegal street drugs. They want to go back home, and they've gotten in terrible trouble. These are people with no criminal record usually. They come here and they just start cycling through the courts and developing serious health problems along with the addictions as well."

———

Indigenous Canadians have been hit particularly hard during the opioid crisis. I wanted to understand why, and what's being done to help.

Shelda Kastor, who is 55 years old and living in the Downtown Eastside, is from the Ochapowace Nation, part of the Cree First Nation. "I was born in Saskatchewan," she told me. "My parents kept me till I was 18 months old before I got scooped, and then I went through living hell until I got adopted, two weeks before I turned seven."

As a toddler, Kastor was one of thousands of Indigenous children taken from their homes as a result of child welfare policies established in the 1960s. These racist policies involved transferring Indigenous children to typically white homes, in some cases relocating them to other provinces or countries without their parents' consent.

The "Sixties Scoop," as it's known, represents a shameful period of Canadian history, one that Kastor and others say hasn't really ended. Indeed, Statistics Canada data reveals that although Indigenous people comprise 4.3% of Canada's population, almost half (48.1%) of all children 14 years and under in foster care are Indigenous. Moreover, compared with only 0.3% of non-Indigenous children, almost 4% of all Indigenous kids are in foster care.

"I'm surprised I even made it," Kastor said. "I'm surprised I'm as sane as I am. I couldn't do anything about it then, but I sure the hell can now. I'm a real little fighter," she added with a grin. "I was adopted by a well-off white family. I was always the only Native, and I was always so ashamed. I always had to fight."

"Do you know anything about your birth parents?" I asked.

"I do, actually. I have an unbelievable memory, and I've always known my real birth name, which is totally blacked out on my adoption papers. I just sort of got into contact with my tribe, and the chief said my real mom is still alive. Apparently she tried to phone here once, but she didn't leave a number, so I couldn't call her. Meanwhile, while that happened, my son died. He didn't get to meet his grandmum."

Today, Kastor is a board member and secretary of the Western Aboriginal Harm Reduction Society (WAHRS), which has about 300 members and operates out of the Vancouver Area Network of Drug Users (VANDU) headquarters on East Hastings Street. When I went to meet her there a huge lineup of people were outside, filling the main entrance. I assumed it was for a free meal or something, which is a common sight in the Downtown Eastside. I didn't want to look as if I were jumping the queue, so Kastor managed to wiggle through the mass of people to find me on the sidewalk outside, her eyeglasses pushed up on top of her long dark hair. I was surprised when she told me that everyone was there for a weekly education meeting. I felt guilty about the assumptions I'd made.

"We're the only Aboriginal harm-reduction group in the entire world," said Kastor. "The other thing I like to say is we're the newest tribe, because we're all products of residential schools or the Sixties Scoop. We're Natives from all over. We're just trying to find our way. We basically lost our culture, and because we've been discriminated against and everything like that for years, it's a way of bonding together. One of the main things is to empower our people and have a voice.

"There's underlying issues why people use to begin with—you don't just go 'Yeah, I want to use drugs.' It's to stop the pain, especially for Native people. Not only the pain from residential schools or the Sixties Scoop; it's everything about losing their family. They thought their parents deserted them when they got scooped. They couldn't figure out why their parents didn't come get 'em. And then the parents felt bad because they let the kids get scooped.

"We have our 'One Heart' healing circle," Kastor told me. "It's just a circle—there's two facilitators, there's an Elder. You can talk about whatever you want, like what's hurting you. They're very, very powerful. A lot of crying, a lot of laughter. People just love being there.

"We need healing, especially with the opioid crisis going on."

Data from the First Nations Health Authority shows that although Indigenous people comprise 3.4% of the population in British Columbia, they account for 10% of all illicit drug overdose deaths and 14% of all overdose events in the province. "Indigenous people are disproportionally represented in people who overdose, people who are addicted, people who die," said Dr. Bonnie Henry, BC's chief medical officer.

"People who are self-declared as First Nations were three times more likely to die of an illicit drug overdose than non–First Nations British Columbians," confirmed Andy Watson with the BC Coroners Service.

What's driving such disproportionate numbers?

"Many of the roots of the problems are related to colonization and intergenerational trauma and lack of community and culture supports," said Dr. Henry. The horrific legacy of the residential school system is continuing to be felt today in many ways. Indigenous youth who had a parent attend residential school have an increased risk of substance use. Indeed, intergenerational trauma can be a huge driver of substance use. So instead of blaming Indigenous people for using illicit drugs, we should be taking a look in the mirror at how our country has directly caused their precipitating trauma in the first place.

"I think it's a very complex picture," said Dr. Shannon McDonald, acting chief medical officer with the First Nations Health Authority. "We have a pain problem, not just a drug problem. Many individuals with histories of trauma, with histories of poverty, with histories of being dealt with in our systemic racist society are more likely to be in the category of somebody who needs help, who needs support. And instead they're often pushed away, labelled, and poorly treated when it comes time to access healthcare and other services to change that trajectory.

"In working with some of the individuals I've met who have a history of use, they often talk about very painful histories, personally in their family, nation, and the situations of their childhood. For example, many of them have been children in care. Come from abusive situations. The use of opioids, alcohol, and other mood-altering drugs helps them cope with systemic painful situations."

"There's a huge role in trauma in the Indigenous population," said Dr. Joe, who has treated many Indigenous people with substance use disorders over the last several decades. "It's very difficult to digest. They're using substances as a means to take away the pain and, more so, to make a bit of their current life less painful. It's very difficult to hear. It affects a lot of people—not just opioids, but other substances as well."

As I looked more closely at the impact of the opioid crisis on Indigenous people, two other aspects came to the surface. One was gender.

"We saw that four in every five deaths across the province involved males," Andy Watson told me. "Well, in the First Nations communities the number was closer to being equally split [between men and women]."

"The gender flip was surprising to me," said Clayton Pecknold. "We're all scratching our heads on that."

Compared with non-Indigenous women, Indigenous women were eight times more likely to overdose, and five times more likely to die from an illicit drug overdose. "We know that many young Indigenous women have been left without the protections of family and community for different reasons in their lives, and have been victims for much of their history," Dr. McDonald explained. She spoke about how Indigenous women in the Downtown Eastside have been treated as disposable to society, as found by the BC Inquiry into Missing and Murdered Women. "There isn't a lot of value placed on them as human beings in those circumstances. It's quite tragic."

"The rate of Aboriginal girls dying is phenomenal," said Shelda Kastor. "They get used and dumped on from the minute they sort of end up on the street. The dealers, everybody uses the girls. That's one of the reasons Native women go missing so often. They think we're disposable for some reason. We gotta make sure that they know that they are somebody. That they can be somebody. We've started, with money from the city, to do an outreach thing to go and connect with those girls down there. Try and keep our girls safe."

The second aspect that struck me about the opioid crisis as it affects Indigenous communities is social dislocation.

"About 90% of the deaths of status First Nations individuals in the opioid crisis have occurred away from home," said Dr. McDonald. "People who are regularly using opioids often have trouble accessing those drugs in their communities and have left home in order to sustain that habit."

Many Indigenous communities have grappled with alcohol abuse for a very long time. The dominant treatment model has been abstinence. However, as we've seen, opioid use disorder is a very different condition—one in which abstinence actually increases the risk of an overdose death when a relapse occurs.

"There are practical things, in that the response to alcohol in First Nations communities in particular has always been very much an abstinence-based program, and it's been a challenge to talk about addictions to opioids and how that's not necessarily the best approach," said Dr. Henry.

Given the intergenerational trauma experienced in many Indigenous communities, combined with the substantially fewer resources
and supports available, it's no wonder that the opioid crisis has been
so devastating. It's clear that any plan to deal with the crisis has to
prioritize responding directly to their needs.

– 8 –

CAN WE PROSECUTE
OUR WAY OUT?

"It was a dark and stormy night," began Oren Bick, senior counsel with the Public Prosecution Service of Canada. I couldn't help laughing.

"It literally was," said Bick, describing the evening of November 29, 2010.

It felt like old times back in law school when we'd talk about the latest criminal case. But this time around Bick was the lead prosecutor on the file. No more training wheels.

"There was snow falling and the police got a call from a tipster telling them that there was a suspicious hiker in the area. Now, these are hiking trails, but they're effectively smuggling trails."

"Do you know the Columbia Valley?"

I shook my head.

"There's walls of mountains on both sides, on the east and on the west, and there's farms all around," he explained, painting a picture of the area south of Chilliwack, BC, some 100 kilometres east of Vancouver. The lush valley spans an uncontrolled section of the Canada–U.S. border. "Along the bottom of each side of the valley are trails that skirt through the woods, along the ridge line. And the police in that area know them well."

Given the time of year, the horrible weather conditions, and history of these trails as cross-border drug-smuggling routes, the RCMP responded to the anonymous tip that night by deploying three officers—one to stake out each of the three trailheads into which the valley would funnel the mysterious hiker.

"In retrospect, that was a strategic error," Bick went on. "It left each officer on his or her own. You know, on a very dark night, basically staking out these three trailheads.

"One officer parked his vehicle on the side of the road. He rolled down his window a crack and just waited. And nothing happened, sitting in his car for about an hour. All of a sudden—and this is a very remote area—another car pulls in right next to him with its headlights on." Before the officer could do anything a man emerged from the trailhead, his body illuminated by the headlights. It was the hiker the police were waiting for. "He was probably, in retrospect, waiting there awhile and was just waiting for his ride to show up," said Bick. It was a dangerous situation for the lone RCMP officer. Alone in the middle of nowhere and outnumbered with no backup, it must have felt like an ambush.

Brazenly, the hiker walked right through the path of the headlights and got into the waiting red Ford Taurus that had pulled up. "So the police officer jumps out and is able to freeze the situation. And, to his credit, he was able to actually arrest both people: the man who had just come out of the woods and the driver."

The officer called for backup, and the two other RCMP officers staking out the other trailheads, five to ten minutes away, came racing to help.

"When the first police car comes, in its headlights they now see a backpack on the ground," said Bick. "The backpack contained 2000 OxyContin pills—which turned out to be fentanyl—a kilogram or two of cocaine, and a small amount of marijuana."

There wasn't enough evidence to charge the driver, Leno Pedro, a one-legged Portuguese man who lived in East Vancouver. The hiker, Andrew Bainbridge, was charged with three counts of possession of illicit drugs for the purpose of trafficking. It was the first illicit fentanyl trafficking prosecution in BC, and is remarkable for having predated the opioid crisis declaration by more than five years.

The one-day trial took place on April 20, 2015. The key issue was whether Bick could prove beyond a reasonable doubt that the backpack of illegal drugs belonged to Bainbridge, whom the Crown alleged was a cross-border drug courier.

There was a problem, however. In the confusion of trying to arrest the two suspects, the RCMP officer who'd staked out the trailhead was unable to say whether he saw Bainbridge actually wearing or carrying the backpack.

"My argument was that, given the situation, the remote area, the only reasonable inference would have been that the backpack had been dropped by the hiker," said Bick. Given the evidence, it was the best argument he could make. "The judge didn't buy that, and he acquitted."

Although Bick respected the judge's verdict, I could tell that, to this day, a few things bothered him about the case.

"The fentanyl didn't make sense to the drug expert," he said. "He had no idea why anybody would be bringing in these fake Oxy pills from the U.S. to Canada, where there were real Oxy pills available in Canada. He thought it might be a price thing.

"Nobody knew really what fentanyl was, aside from some of the medical literature that was out there. Nobody from the police had seen it. The drug expert who was brought in to look at it had never seen it used as a street drug in that form at that time. Since then, about 2012, 2013, 2014, we saw a flood of it."

The Bainbridge prosecution was indeed a harbinger of what was to come. But there was another twist in the case that would come back to haunt the authorities.

Back on that dark and stormy night in 2010, after the police had arrested Bainbridge the hiker and Pedro the driver, they released them both from police custody without any conditions. The RCMP put a tail on the two men—a covert team to follow each one. The plan was to further the investigation by seeing what they'd do next and who they'd meet with. After all, a goal in every drug trafficking case is to move up the chain as far as possible in order to identify and prosecute those with the greatest culpability.

Bainbridge, a thirtysomething Indigenous man, simply returned to his home in Richmond to be with his wife and two-year-old son. That police tail failed to generate anything of use. Pedro, however, left the police station and drove straight to the Knight & Day Restaurant on Loughheed Highway and Boundary Road in Vancouver. The all-day breakfast diner is located right beside the TransCanada Highway. It's also 750 metres from the new Vancouver Police Department (VPD) building that was under construction at the time. Maybe he was just hungry after his late-night rendezvous and run-in with police?

Pedro made a call from a payphone at the restaurant. "It's 2010, so there's still payphones around," Bick reminded me. Pedro then sat down in a booth at the diner. "Fifteen minutes later, who shows up but a guy named Walter McCormick, who was known to the police at that time," said Bick. McCormick had three prior drug trafficking–related convictions, including one in Seattle, Washington, for conspiracy to distribute cocaine from Canada to the United States. McCormick had been sentenced to 10 years imprisonment in the U.S., but as a Canadian citizen he was allowed to transfer to Canada to serve his time. Our jails aren't as harsh, and our parole is easier to get.

"They investigated a bit but they couldn't really get anywhere," explained Bick. "About five years later I would be prosecuting Walter McCormick in the biggest fentanyl bust the VPD ever did."

———

It was October 2014, in the midst of a surge of illicit drug overdose deaths in BC. The VPD was investigating an individual they suspected of selling "bad heroin" (heroin laced with illicit fentanyl) in the Downtown Eastside.

Undercover officers quickly advanced their investigation to the point where they were able to buy 1000 fentanyl pills from a mid-level drug supplier (Raymon Ranu) on January 8, 2015, for $11,000. Unbeknownst to Ranu the bills were traceable, and the police had him under surveillance. They wanted to know who was supplying him with the illicit fentanyl that was killing a growing number of people. Both before and after the transaction, police observed Ranu meeting with none other than Walter McCormick. They'd need more evidence if they were going to nab him, though. Now McCormick was in their dragnet.

About a week later, McCormick supplied Ranu with another 1000 fentanyl pills that Ranu again sold to the undercover officer. Ten days after that, the same thing happened. On February 4, 2015, a fourth transaction for more illicit fentanyl was arranged, with Ranu again as the middleman between McCormick and the undercover officer—this time for 2000 fentanyl pills. Police believed they had McCormick.

On February 17, 2015, they arrested McCormick. He had two cell phones, $1205 in cash, and a key to a storage locker on him. Police searched his vehicle, home, and the storage locker. They unearthed a veritable treasure trove of illicit drugs and firearms:

- 27,000 fentanyl pills
- 4.054 kilograms of cocaine
- 1.016 kilograms of methamphetamine
- 374 grams of MDMA

- 5 grams of heroin
- 22.56 kilograms of cannabis
- 3 kilograms of cannabis resin
- 92,833 alprazolam pills (Xanax)
- $171,905 in cash
- 600,000 pills that weren't controlled drugs under the Controlled Drugs and Substance Act
- 4.54 kilograms of cutting agents
- 44 kilograms of excipients and dyes (commonly used as fillers and dyes in pills and tablets)
- a Heckler & Koch USP .40-calibre pistol, with readily accessible ammunition
- a .22-calibre rifle

They'd nabbed a big fish: the street value of the illicit drugs seized was $2.03 million. It would have been an arduous process sifting through this mountain of evidence, but investigators were meticulous. They went through the seized cash and found that McCormick was in possession of a total of $17,200 in traceable bills with which the undercover police officer had paid Ranu for three of the four transactions. They had McCormick dead to rights.

McCormick was released on bail two days after his arrest and started living in a series of apartments and hotels. His relationship with his common-law partner, whom he'd been with for over a decade, ended.

"McCormick is an example of someone who is at the top of the chain, although I can't prove to what extent he was involved in importing," said Bick. "We do know that at the time he was caught he was distributing at a very high level, high volume."

Just 15 months later, on May 18, 2016, while still on bail and awaiting trial, McCormick was at it again. After he refused to be evicted from the Sandman Hotel in Richmond, the hotel manager found evidence of illegal drugs and called the police. They located McCormick outside, hiding in a UPS truck. He was severely intoxicated with drugs and alcohol. They seized 1000 fentanyl pills, two kilograms of cocaine, 18.1 kilograms of marijuana, 4285 alprazolam pills, and $4736 cash from his vehicle, his hotel room, and the parking lot outside his room. McCormick was charged on June 24, 2016, and was detained pending trial.

He pleaded guilty to a range of trafficking charges. At the time of sentencing, he was 53 years old. The court heard that McCormick was born in Kelowna, BC; that his mother died when he was six and so he was raised by his father. He had a grade 12 education and had been employed as an iron worker for about 22 years. His lawyer said he had problems with drugs and alcohol. He'd had a tough life.

The maximum penalty for trafficking in drugs like heroin, cocaine, and fentanyl is life imprisonment, but it's rare to see sentences beyond 10 years in Canada, except for importation and large-scale criminal conspiracies. Bick called for McCormick to be given 18 years' imprisonment—an "exemplary sentence for an exemplary case" to recognize the harm that fentanyl was causing in the community. Defence counsel asked for a prison sentence of eight to nine years.

"Mr. McCormick was the supplier to a mid-level drug trafficker. He was three levels removed from the level of a street trafficker," said Judge Bonnie Craig of the BC Provincial Court on January 30, 2017, in sentencing him. "Mr. McCormick was the principal actor; he was not acting as a courier or a middle-man. He controlled his operation.

"I recognize that a sentence above any established range will not lead to an end to the fentanyl epidemic," Judge Craig went on. "The lure of substantial profit for lower risk, with the awareness of the very real and substantial risk to life that comes from trafficking in fentanyl must be counteracted with the threat of a significant jail sentence on conviction."

Judge Craig sentenced McCormick to 14 years' imprisonment.

It's not just high-level fentanyl traffickers like Walter McCormick who are receiving stiff sentences by the courts. Street-level distributors who sell to end users are also being hit. That includes dealers who walk around or use bikes to sell drugs in particularly concentrated geographic areas. Others run dial-a-dope operations that take orders by cell phone and deliver illicit drugs to the purchaser's home or another provided address. "Crack shacks" are fixed locations where drugs can be purchased, but are less common since they're easier for police to locate and shut down.

In *R. v. Smith*, the BC Court of Appeal held in a landmark 2017 decision that street-level dealers convicted of fentanyl trafficking should receive more stringent sentences too, typically within the range of 18 to 36 months' imprisonment. This is at least triple the starting point for street-level heroin trafficking, which is six months in jail.

"As matters stand today, other dangerous drugs do not kill as frequently, accidentally, or as unpredictably as fentanyl, but the risks posed by those drugs should not be minimized even by comparison with fentanyl," said Justice David Harris in a majority decision of the BC Court of Appeal. "Recognizing a different and markedly higher sentencing range for street-level dealing in fentanyl turns on the enhanced risks associated with that activity and the individual responsibility of dealers given those risks and public knowledge of them."

But who are these street-level fentanyl dealers, and is there any evidence that stiffer sentences will deter them?

———

Just off Hastings and Main in Vancouver's Downtown Eastside is the Hotel Maple, a narrow, eight-storey brick building that's been converted to an 81-unit social housing complex run by PHS Community

Services Society. And the alleyway behind the Hotel Maple, like many others in the area, is where illicit drugs are bought and sold.

"One of our staff, a peer employee, got called out to the alley to help an overdose," said Jennifer Breakspear, executive director of PHS. When the staff member came outside they saw an individual lying on the ground while someone else was doing rescue breathing, trying to revive them.

"I just sold this to her," said the man doing the rescue breathing. "Did I kill her?"

"He had sold the person the drugs and was helping her inject," said Breakspear. "He was really upset. He was doing what he needed to do. He's not a bad guy. He's caught up in it as much as the person who used it."

The street-level dealer had stayed to try to save his customer's life despite the legal risk he was putting himself in. He could have been criminally charged with trafficking or worse if the person had died. Breakspear's story broke the stereotypical mould in my mind about what these dealers were: heartless individuals whose only motivation in life was money.

"I think we need to treat the street-level folks with as much compassion as we're treating the folks that are buying from them. They don't have an option. Life has led them to a point where their options are so limited, and we're seeing this," said Breakspear.

Many people I spoke with—including criminal defence lawyers, criminologists, healthcare professionals, and people who use drugs—argued that the weight of enforcement against fentanyl traffickers has largely fallen on street-level dealers who are often dealing to support their own addiction, and that big prosecutions like the McCormick case are actually few and far between.

"It would be nice if they actually got somebody who really fit trafficking," said Mark Gervin, a criminal defence lawyer and director of legal services with UBC's Indigenous Community Legal Clinic. "I mean at best, in a great year, they get a small amount of mid-level people who aren't dealing for drugs. They're having zero effect on anything. Most of what we see—the trafficking or the possession for the purpose of trafficking in the Downtown Eastside—those people are told, 'You go and sell 10 whatever, come back, and we'll give you some heroin or fentanyl.'"

I wanted to know whether there was any hard data to confirm or deny these claims, either in reported court cases or in police files. Haley Hrymak is a criminal lawyer who took a leave of absence from her job to pursue her Master of Laws through researching the opioid crisis at UBC, which is where I met her. Hrymak dug into all the reported sentencing decisions for street-level fentanyl traffickers in BC between January 1, 2016, and November 1, 2017, to learn more about these individuals and how the courts are dealing with them. She found that of the 14 street-level fentanyl traffickers sentenced during this period, only two weren't current or former drug users.

"Addiction motivated nearly all the individuals who were engaging in street-level trafficking," writes Hrymak. "Addiction is a disease that involves engaging in drug use on an ongoing basis despite risk of harm or negative consequences associated with these behaviours. Research shows that the threat of an increased jail term does not dissolve an addiction."

I also wanted to ask the Vancouver Police Department about these claims, but before I did, I tracked down a copy of the VPD's Drug Policy statement. It reads, in part: "Within the context of enforcement, street-level drug trafficking remains a priority. This includes the 'addicted trafficker' as well as the 'non-addicted trafficker.' The VPD will not distinguish between the two; however, enforcement will be directed more at traffickers who exhibit a higher degree of organization and coordination."

"I haven't seen a lot of charges publicly for non-street-level traffickers, people who are mid or higher up in the chain. Is that a fair perception?" I asked.

"That's a fair perception," said Deputy Chief Constable Laurence Rankin with the VPD. "We've had some success with the drug forces operation over the last year, where we've identified and been able to target and successfully charge individuals that are trafficking in firearms and fentanyl, but again, I think it's lost in just the everyday."

I asked Rankin for statistics on trafficking prosecutions over the last few years to get a better idea of what's happening on the front lines of policing during the opioid crisis in Vancouver. It took organized crime analysts about a month to crunch the numbers.

Between 2015 and 2017, the VPD filed a total of 899 illicit drug trafficking charges (which includes trafficking and possession for the purposes of trafficking). By May 2018, these charges had resulted in a total of 160 convictions, representing 17.8% of charges.

"Yeah, that's a low conviction rate," said Inspector Bill Spearn with the VPD. "A lot of those charges would be recommended; some of them may go through to conviction; they may not get charge approval; the charges may get stayed. A lot of these people would go through diversion in the drug courts and plead to possession in order to get into the drug courts and go into that program, even though we recommended possession for the purposes of trafficking or trafficking. Because they pled to possession, they wouldn't show up in here as a conviction."

How many of these charges involved mid- to high-level traffickers versus street-level dealers? It turned out that it isn't possible to know for sure without the VPD doing a time-consuming case-by-case review. But it was possible to get a rough idea by breaking it down into those cases dealt with by ordinary patrol units (which typically deal with street-level dealers) versus the VPD Organized Crime Section, which runs projects targeting major trafficking operations.

Only 31 out of 899 (3.4%) of drug trafficking charges in Vancouver between 2015 and 2017 were mid/high-level traffickers targeted by the VPD Organized Crime Section. As of May 2018, only six of these individuals had been convicted (from one project in 2015).

"The complexity of those files is much greater," said Inspector Spearn. "Just about all of them are still in the court system. It's just a slow process, as you know, to get them through the court system."

So the data seemed to back up what I'd been hearing from critics: it's the street-level dealers who are overwhelmingly the ones being charged. Since drug trafficking is hierarchical, there are a lot more people at the bottom, and these individuals are also the most visible and easiest to catch. It's the charging and conviction of mid- to high-level fentanyl traffickers that are the exception. A similar phenomenon exists in the United States, which has the highest per capita rates of incarceration of anywhere in the world.

"Well, in the United States the problem is that we seem to be incredibly successful at arresting and incarcerating people who are at the retail end and not the wholesale or the manufacturing end," said Dr. Richard Frank. "And here that causes as many problems as it solves. You now have a group of people who, if they weren't hard-core criminals at the beginning—they're just selling drugs—they go to prison and sharpen their trade there. They're often traumatized there, and then in the U.S. your chances of being employed are dramatically reduced on the way out, and your chances of having other kinds of problems are increased as well. So obviously the net effect is not all that positive."

Indeed, as then Chief Justice Antonio Lamer of the Supreme Court of Canada recognized in a 2000 judgment, "Prison has been characterized by some as a finishing school for criminals and as ill-preparing them for reintegration into society."

"One of the reasons we see so many street-level traffickers being prosecuted is because the number of man hours it takes the police end to do that is so much less," said Oren Bick. "It's exponentially less than the amount of man hours it will take to successfully investigate a higher-level trafficker who is not putting himself out there on the street every day—not exposing himself.

"Sometimes it's easier to achieve mandates by focusing on the low-hanging fruit," Bick continued. "They have a number of goals, annual performance reviews, just like the rest of us do, and they want to be seen as doing something. And to the extent that they're taking the lower-level trafficker off the street, that's still a good result—and it's a lot easier in terms of man hours than addressing someone who is higher up on the chain.

"If the police do get more resources to focus more time on higher-level cases, that would be good. The problem is that you don't always see the results. If a unit that investigates high-level drug traffickers closes only four or five files a year, then the results might not be enough to justify the money in the view of the people who allocate that kind of money."

———

I wanted to understand whether there were any unique challenges in prosecuting fentanyl trafficking cases, so I asked Bick.

"From a prosecution point of view, prosecuting fentanyl cases is the same as prosecuting any other drug case," he told me. "You have to prove the possession, the control, the knowledge. That sort of thing.

"There's unique challenges from the police point of view. The police have a lot of pressures on them that contradict each other. They've got a lot of pressure on them not to let fentanyl hit the streets. They don't want to be accused of jeopardizing lives in an effort to further their investigation, which differs from the attitude that police have had traditionally for other drugs.

"I've seen [cocaine] cases, I've prosecuted them, where police sit and watch and watch and watch and wait, and more cocaine is being delivered and being delivered and being delivered, and the police are gathering evidence as they're watching where every delivery goes, and that sort of thing. It ends up being a solid case to prosecute because the police have seen the same thing happen three or four times, and so there's a strong case against the person who does it.

"With fentanyl, there's counter-pressure to end investigations early in order to avoid fentanyl hitting the streets, which makes for a less compelling prosecution, or a prosecution of the arguably less culpable person in the organization.

"There's always a point in the police investigation where they need to decide when they're pulling the trigger. Do they wait for another few packages to go by in order to make their grounds to search the destination of the package stronger, or do they conduct more surveillance to see who is receiving the packages?"

Bick's explanation was compelling. It offered another reason why we see so few kingpins being prosecuted for fentanyl trafficking, something that one of my RCMP sources confirmed.

Fentanyl really has been a game changer for law enforcement. Given its toxicity, the police can't let an illicit pipeline like that continue to flow while they work their way up the trafficking food chain—which is why many investigations never get much further than a street-level dealer. And there's always someone willing to take their place once they're arrested.

———

On the surface, there was nothing all that special about Barrett Richard Jordan's case. But today every judge, Crown prosecutor, and criminal defence lawyer in the country knows his name.

Jordan was arrested in December 2008 and eventually charged along with 10 others for his role in running a dial-a-dope operation in the BC Lower Mainland. The Crown prosecutor had to ask for more time to present the "mountain of evidence" against him at the preliminary inquiry before his trial.

Jordan was convicted in February 2013 but appealed his case all the way up to the Supreme Court of Canada. He wasn't arguing that he was innocent. Instead, his lawyers argued his "right to be tried within a reasonable time" under the Canadian Charter of Rights and Freedoms was violated because of excessive delay. It had taken just over four years (49.5 months) from the time he was charged to the end of his trial. Although accused people are presumed innocent, many languish for long periods of time in pre-trial detention. In some provinces, there are more people in custody awaiting trial than have actually been convicted. And drawn-out prosecutions can also be harmful to victims.

While the trial judge and BC Court of Appeal rejected Jordan's Charter claim, the Supreme Court allowed his appeal in July 2016. It overturned his drug trafficking convictions and entered a stay of proceedings. Jordan was a free man.

"As we have observed, a culture of complacency towards delay has emerged in the criminal justice system," said Justices Moldaver, Karakatsanis, and Brown for the majority. "Unnecessary procedures and adjournments, inefficient practices, and inadequate institutional resources are accepted as the norm and give rise to ever-increasing delay. This culture of delay 'causes great harm to public confidence in the justice system.' It 'rewards the wrong behaviour, frustrates the well-intentioned, makes frequent users of the system cynical and disillusioned, and frustrates the rehabilitative goals of the system.'"

These judges set a general deadline of 18 months for cases in provincial court and 30 months for cases in superior court (which hears only some serious charges). If it takes longer than that from the charge date to the end of trial, it's presumed that the rights of the accused have been violated. There are some exceptions for defence delays and exceptional circumstances, but *R. v. Jordan* sets a "best before" date after which prosecutions are at risk of being turfed out, no matter how grave the case. Murder, sexual offences against kids, drug trafficking cases—such charges have since been tossed out because of *Jordan*.

"*Jordan* has really, really slowed us down as to how we can respond. It's really put a strain on our resources. It's probably the biggest change in policing I've ever seen in my career," said Inspector Spearn. "Let's say we arrest somebody for drug trafficking. We can't even lay a charge until we get all the drugs analyzed, you know, get full disclosure up front, because if we lay a charge, then our *Jordan* clock starts ticking and we can run into a lot of issues.

"If we arrest a fentanyl dealer, we can't even hold them in custody. So we release them so that we can do all our disclosure—and they just go back out on the street and sell more drugs and kill more people."

Inspector Spearn's concerns aren't merely theoretical. An alleged fentanyl dealer in Ontario recently had his charges stayed because of the *Jordan* decision. He walked out of the courtroom a free man, without any trial.

———

Even if police and prosecutors are able to navigate all the pitfalls and perils of prosecuting a fentanyl trafficker, will stiff jail terms have any impact in stemming the opioid crisis?

"If you were to scoop up 100% of them today, that would be filled with another group of people," said Mark Gervin, explaining that every time a fentanyl dealer is arrested, another is easily recruited to take their place. "I mean it's all about the demand.

"They're not reading newspapers. They're not reading case law. They're not talking to people who are doing the sentences. So they have no idea what's going on. I would talk to the first-timers and they'd say, 'Well, I was just told that we'd get six months' probation.' So they're being lied to. They're in for a shock."

Although the police officers I interviewed all conceded that trying to crack down on the supply of illicit opioids isn't going to solve the crisis, they argued that there's a need to pursue those who are trafficking illicit fentanyl.

"I can tell you that I have spoken to drug dealers who won't deal fentanyl because they don't want to go to jail for eight years or ten years, where they used to be worried about going to jail for six months or a year," said Staff Sergeant Conor King with the Victoria Police Department. "They won't deal fentanyl anymore. Is it working every time? I guess probably not. Is it working sometimes? Yes, it is. It's the structure we've got right now and nothing else."

But other police officers seemed less optimistic about the impact of prosecuting traffickers.

"You feel like the little Dutch boy putting your finger in a dike, but at the same time we have enough information to move on any number of files," said Deputy Chief Constable Laurence Rankin. "At the end of the day, we're taking individuals off the street that are extremely violent, that are engaged in extremely violent behaviour and happen to be dealing fentanyl."

"We've had some good successes in the last year and a half, hitting traffickers that are specifically targeting the high-risk areas," said Dwayne McDonald, Assistant Commissioner and officer in charge of the Surrey RCMP detachment. "But, like anything, as soon as you take one out, there's a vacuum and it's filled almost instantly by somebody else."

Both Rankin and McDonald seemed to be conceding that we should have little expectation of prosecuting our way out of the opioid crisis.

"You've probably talked to people who do doubt it, that higher sentences deter. I think where people get a bit sidetracked is that they don't deter everyone," said Bick. "If somebody is saying that high sentences universally deter, then that's wrong. There will always be someone who is willing to take up the mantle no matter how high the potential sentence is, but generally deterrence can also be seen as at least deterring some segment of the population from engaging in this type of activity."

Bick's comments gave me pause, reminding me that there's a ton of research on whether stiffer penalties actually deter crime or not.

"Research shows clearly that the chance of being caught is a vastly more effective deterrent than even draconian punishment," concluded the U.S. National Institute of Justice (NIJ) in a summary of the available criminology research. "Laws and policies designed to deter crime by focusing mainly on increasing the severity of punishment are ineffective partly because criminals know little about the sanctions for specific crimes. More severe punishments do not 'chasten' individuals convicted of crimes, and prisons may exacerbate recidivism (re-offending)."

"Effective policing that leads to swift and certain (but not necessarily severe) sanctions is a better deterrent than the threat of incarceration," found the NIJ. Interestingly, legal sanctions also have less of a deterrent effect on serious offences (including "hard-drug" trafficking) than on minor, non-violent crimes.

Despite this evidence, President Donald Trump has gone so far as to propose that fentanyl traffickers be subject to the death penalty. It turns out that there is no proof that even the death penalty deters criminals.

What's generally needed to deter people from engaging in criminal behaviour is a greater certainty of being caught and then swiftly punished. On both of those counts, the current situation with fentanyl trafficking falls hopelessly short. The probability of a fentanyl manufacturer, importer, or high-level trafficker being arrested is incredibly low, and there are big delays in meting out punishment. And if we're talking about a street-level addicted fentanyl dealer, the threat of criminal sanctions is even less likely to deter them.

"We're not arresting our way out of this one," conceded Deputy Chief Serr. "I've been around the world of drug enforcement for a long time. We have never, to date, ever stopped a drug trend, whether it be crack cocaine, cocaine, heroin, or methamphetamine. Every one of those drugs is still readily available.

"We've done a large seizure, which is fantastic and what we need to do, but all we've done is, for a short period of time, change the market of that drug. The price may have gone up and it may be a little harder to find, but we've never eradicated a drug."

But even that temporary effect has been questioned. Street-level data after major drug busts challenges the idea that enforcement efforts actually have any noticeable impact on drug prices and availability.

"Our data suggest that drug prices on the city's streets have been unaffected by law enforcement efforts," found a report by the BC Centre for Excellence in HIV/AIDS. "Specifically, annual street-level data suggest the price of heroin, cocaine, crack cocaine and crystal methamphetamine have remained low and stable, placing doubt on assertions by the Royal Canadian Mounted Police that interdiction efforts have had an impact on the availability of illicit drugs at the street level."

I also heard a concern that I hadn't anticipated—one that was raised separately by two different groups representing people who use drugs.

"We've heard tons of complaints about police just taking drug dealers' drugs and money. Basically, just letting them go," said Westfall. "When the cops do that it just makes the drug market more dangerous for people, because now they can't go to their guy. They have to go somewhere else, and they have to find out if their drugs are safe or not. Sometimes they're not."

———

When I met with Staff Sergeant King in his Victoria office, I couldn't help noticing the large "targeting" chart on his wall. It looked like a scene from the HBO television series *The Wire*. The chart showed known and suspected drug traffickers, with lines connecting them to each other. There were, of course, several "Mr. X" figures with no names or no photos—people whom the police had yet to identify but knew were players in the importation and trafficking network.

"The goal is to investigate them, get their evidence, get charges on them, and get convictions," said King, who was sporting a goatee and wore a pressed business shirt with a police-issue semi-automatic black matte Glock handgun holstered on his leather belt.

He noted that one of their recent convictions for fentanyl trafficking had netted a 12-year prison sentence. But King is under no illusions about what he and his policing colleagues are up against. "Well, I'm not entirely sure that what we're doing is working, because our sole goal is to stop overdose deaths," he conceded.

King and all the other law enforcement and border officials I spoke with were clearly dedicated to their work. They were committed to doing what they could to address the opioid crisis. But they also frankly admitted to me, to varying degrees, that trying to have any major impact on the opioid crisis by waging a war on the supply of illicit fentanyl is not going to work. Period.

With a synthetic drug like fentanyl that can be made anywhere on the planet, it's all the more impossible to stamp out the supply. Add the dark web, cryptocurrencies, and a lack of legal tools to the mix, and you've got a seemingly insurmountable task.

"Am I a believer that we're going to be able to turn off the tap of illicit fentanyl?" King asked. "We haven't been able to turn off the tap of cocaine or heroin for 60 years."

— 9 —

WHAT IS NALOXONE
AND IS IT THE SOLUTION?

Any other time a regular citizen saved 148 lives, they'd be in the national news and get a medal from the Governor General. We'd all know their name. A school, park, or city street would probably get named after them too.

Surrey's 135A Street—known locally as "the strip"—is a place few Canadians have heard of. On any given night in early 2018, there were 80 to 90 tents with 90 to 140 people living in them on this derelict side street that's about 40 minutes from downtown Vancouver. Nearby there's a corner store, a thrift shop, a pawnbroker, fast food restaurants, a food bank, and some low-rent hotels. The homeless residents of this tent city, which stretched for three blocks, included people with mental health and substance use issues. The RCMP got involved because of increasing property crime in the area and violent crimes being committed against these vulnerable homeless people.

"The violence in that community from drug dealers was huge, it was astronomical," said Inspector Shawna Baher with the Surrey RCMP detachment. Among other responsibilities, she heads up the drug section, criminal intelligence section, and gang task force as well as the auto crime and property crime units. Talk about having a lot on your plate at work. Baher has short, straight brown hair and has worked undercover. I've met other undercover officers before and, like Baher, you'd never know they were cops if you saw them on the street.

"What kind of offences were you seeing at 135A Street?" I asked her.

"Beatings, stabbings, robberies, a lot of intimidation, sexual assault on females."

I met Baher and her boss, Assistant Commissioner Dwayne McDonald, at the Surrey RCMP headquarters, just across the street from the busy provincial courthouse. McDonald, who has 26 years of policing experience, was promoted in November 2016 to officer in charge of the Surrey RCMP—essentially the chief of police. Nothing could have quite prepared him for taking on that role in the midst of the opioid crisis. Seeing the rising overdose death count across Surrey and the ongoing crime happening on 135A Street, McDonald and his team had to try something different.

"We developed the Surrey Outreach Team," he told me. "We basically placed 16 regular RCMP members in a portable office, for lack of a better word, or trailer, and we've partnered with Fraser Health, with BC Housing, with bylaws, and with the Front Room [a non-profit community agency]. Our main mandate in that area is to develop relationships with the people there, try and help them transition from 135A to housing, to treatment, to rehab, to anywhere other than having to be homeless."

When McDonald arrived, the situation on the strip was downright dystopian.

"People would be vacating their bowels in buckets in tents and then just throwing them out on the street," he said. "We put in some bathrooms. Well, I think we've gone through two service providers already who have refused now to continue because it's so filthy. In agreement with the City and bylaws, we'll go in every morning and do a cleanup. Everyone brings out their junk and stuff they don't want anymore. Everyone will take their tents down and we'll power wash the street every two weeks now, just because it's necessary.

"We'll do a tent count and a person count every day, usually at night. Last night we had 82 tents. The number of people sleeping in tents were 115, and I think there was maybe one arrest because of a fight."

Another purpose of the Surrey Outreach Team's daily walk-around is to get to know people on the strip, especially newcomers, and try to direct them to services. Peer-based support is also part of 135A Street.

And given the massive number of overdoses in the area, naloxone, which can reverse an opioid overdose, has been handed out widely. "With the advent of the use of naloxone and the fact that, especially in some of the higher-risk areas, it's provided free to the clients, we find out that a lot of them are reviving each other and aren't calling police, fire, or ambulance," said McDonald. The widespread free distribution of naloxone to the residents of 135A Street is credited with saving countless lives.

One person living there even took it upon himself to help out.

"We had one guy, what was his name? Jim," said Inspector Baher. "He was a homeless guy, and he rode his bicycle up and down 135A Street. Doug, that was his name. Just driving around with a little take-home naloxone kit and administering it. You have people like that, who are taking responsibility. He's not only educating. He's out there helping people, and he's trying to do it from that grassroots movement."

I wanted to find out more about Doug.

Coincidentally, as I was doing some further research, I visited the BC Centre for Disease Control's naloxone website (www.towardtheheart .com). At the bottom of the page was a video about someone named Doug. Could it be the same guy? I clicked on the link.

"They call me 'Little Doug' on the street," said the man in the video. He had a kind, gentle voice. Hazel eyes, a weathered but friendly face. A reddish beard and wavy, shoulder-length hair. "I carry naloxone in Surrey," he said. "Since I was homeless and in that neighbourhood where the demand was, I thought I could do something useful. That's what it's all about, is preventing death.

"Fentanyl is a new addition causing a lot of overdoses. There are no sure ways to reverse an overdose other than naloxone. It's the wonder drug that changes the event."

It turns out that "Little Doug" is Douglas Nickerson. He's the guy Inspector Baher was talking about—the guy driving around 135A Street on his bicycle, saving lives with naloxone all on his own.

All told, Little Doug reversed 148 overdoses. He was honoured with Surrey's "Heart of the City" Award a few days before he died from pancreatic cancer on October 28, 2017. He was 59 years old. I don't know exactly why, but watching him share his story in that video, in his own words, brought tears to my eyes. Maybe it was the small glimmer of hope that I finally saw shining through after weeks of hearing about little else but death and hopelessness.

Little Doug's selfless heroism and gentle humility, all the while himself homeless and having struggled with opioid addiction, were so inspiring. I wish I could have met him while he was alive. I wanted to do something to recognize what he and countless other unsung heroes have done during the opioid crisis, and so that's why I've dedicated this book to his memory. Now you know the name of this hero too.

——

"It's a miracle drug," said Linda Lupini. Naloxone has a remarkable ability to seemingly resurrect people who are barely breathing, or not breathing at all—just a few minutes later they're walking around and talking. That's the reason it's sometimes called the "Lazarus" drug, alluding to the Biblical account of Jesus raising Lazarus from the dead. It's no exaggeration to call it an "antidote" to an opioid overdose.

Naloxone is an "opioid antagonist" medication, meaning that it blocks opiate receptors, temporarily reversing the effects of opioids like fentanyl, heroin, and oxycodone. During an overdose, opioids are telling your brain to breathe less, or to stop breathing altogether. Naloxone works by temporarily stopping those signals, which can be life-threatening. It can take three to five minutes for naloxone to take effect, so overdose victims may need to be given rescue breathing to ensure that enough oxygen is reaching the brain. In serious cases, an overdose victim may go into cardiac arrest and also need CPR. If you don't have naloxone, you can still try to save someone's life by breathing for them and calling 911 until help arrives.

Sold under the brand name Narcan, naloxone is the number one emergency response for keeping people alive during an opioid overdose. For that reason, Health Canada "delisted" naloxone in March 2016, meaning it can now be obtained over the counter, without a prescription.

Naloxone is typically administered through an intra-muscular injection (into the muscle of the arm, thigh, or buttocks) or as a nasal spray. It's safe and can be given by someone who has minimal training—studies have shown naloxone to be 94% effective when administered by laypeople. There are no known negative consequences of giving someone naloxone if they're not, in fact, experiencing an opioid overdose. And there's no potential for it to be abused. So experts say that when someone is exhibiting signs of an overdose and you're unsure whether opioids were the cause, it's still safe to administer naloxone.

The more potent the opioids, the greater the quantity of naloxone may be needed to reverse the overdose. Many overdose victims require several doses in order to be revived. If carfentanyl caused the overdose, it can reportedly take nine to ten naloxone doses to revive someone—and that's several take-home naloxone kits' worth of medication, so one kit wouldn't be enough.

There's something ironic about the fact that naloxone was developed at almost exactly the same time as fentanyl, but on different continents by two different teams of scientists.

"I look at that almost in a weird way—like if we were to believe for a second that there's this kind of yin and yang, as it were, for the universe," said Staff Sergeant Conor King. "Just when fentanyl came along, naloxone had been around for years but it became more widely available, and it's like the two fit together in this weird kind of way."

Indeed, the original patent for naloxone was filed in 1961. Its original aim was to deal with one of the less serious side effects of opioid addiction: constipation. Its inventor, Jack Fishman, had no idea that it would come to save hundreds of thousands of lives during the opioid crisis for its ability to reverse the effects of an opioid overdose. He died in 2013 at the age of 83, never having profited from the life-saving drug he invented because the patent had expired. Tragically, his own stepson died from a heroin overdose in Florida when naloxone was still tightly controlled and hadn't yet been made available to the public.

———

"Someone's down!"

"People would literally be yelling at paramedics," said Lupini. "We had bike paramedics to go through alleys and lanes, and that worked really well because they've got all their equipment with them. Otherwise they're parking, they're running quite a distance with drug kits and all sorts of things."

In the early days of the opioid crisis, as overdose rates skyrocketed, Lupini's ambulance service had to split up paramedic teams to patrol solo on bikes, roving around high-risk areas rather than waiting for

911 calls. The bike paramedics were literally waiting for someone else to drop to the ground, no longer breathing, their skin quickly turning blue.

The first emergency response to the opioid crisis is to keep people alive who have overdosed. Since every second counts during an overdose and naloxone is the antidote, it must be freely available and widely distributed anywhere an overdose has occurred or is likely to occur. People need to be trained and know how to administer it during an emergency. That training is available for free online at www.naloxonetraining.com and takes only 10 to 15 minutes.

In addition to all the paramedics, firefighters, and police officers carrying and being trained in how to administer naloxone, it should be widely distributed for free to the general public, including people who use drugs, their families and friends, and people being released from custody. These take-home naloxone kits should also be renewed as they're used or expire. Because of the stigma around drug use and its ongoing criminalization, there can't be any barriers around accessing this lifesaving drug.

A BC Centre for Disease Control study published in *The Lancet Public Health* journal found that the rapid, wide-scale distribution of naloxone kits has prevented even more overdose deaths from occurring in BC. Between January and October 2016, 298 deaths were averted—over a quarter (26%) of all possible overdose-related deaths—by the administration of naloxone by drug users, community organizations, and concerned citizens—people like "Little Doug" Nickerson. Tragically, the same *Lancet* study found that if the take-home naloxone program had been ramped up earlier, an additional 118 lives would likely have been saved.

"People self-report back and say, 'I used my kit. I saved my friend,'" said Inspector Bill Spearn. "Take-home naloxone was probably one of the most successful harm reduction initiatives we've had."

As I walked through the Downtown Eastside to meet with various people for this study, I saw the distinctive kits everywhere I turned, often dangling from backpacks. They look like a black sunglasses case with a zipper, bearing a cross emblazoned with the word "NALOXONE." These kits contain naloxone itself (either in a nasal spray or in ampoule vials with syringes) along with alcohol swabs, protective gloves, a breathing mask for providing mouth-to-mouth resuscitation, and a card describing exactly what to do in the event of an overdose. They're distributed by pharmacies and various organizations, many of which have weekly standing orders for them.

"We are the first first responders," said Shelda Kastor. "We're the ones who keep them alive. Those are our friends, they're people we know." Kastor has personally administered naloxone 14 times to help people who've overdosed.

"The first one is always very scary," she told me. "I was working the window at Washington Needle Depot and somebody came to the window and said, 'We need the kit! We need the kit! Somebody's OD'd.' I was there by myself, so I locked up the place, grabbed the kit, and went running out. Just as I saw the guy, I realized there's a cop car at the end of the alley." She threw the naloxone kit she had at the person who'd come asking for it so that they could get started. "I ran down to the cop and said, 'There's a guy OD'ing! There's a guy OD'ing!' The cop says, 'Go run down to Insite and get a nurse.' I said, 'Are you fricking kidding me?'"

There was no time to get a nurse. Kastor left the police officer and ran back to the person who'd overdosed. She readied a naloxone dose in a syringe for the first time. "When I went to puncture his thigh, I was like 'Oh my God, am I going to go too deep and get him in the bone or something?' It was very scary."

"What happened?" I asked.

"He died.

"They all survived after that. One time it was so cold out my fingers got numb, and I was trying to snap that little vial. And those things can snap and break and can cut your hands, cut your fingers. My fingers were so, so cold I couldn't even snap the thing. All I'm worrying about is, 'I gotta get this open so I can help this person.'"

"The people carry naloxone on the streets, and everyone has their needles out when somebody ends up in a perceived or real overdose event," said Vancouver Fire Chief Darrell Reid. "A lot of times, our crews are finding that the person's received naloxone even before we've arrived a minute later, a minute and a half later. Our specialty in patient management has actually become early management. That's the life-saving skill, more so than the administration of naloxone. It's a real basic resuscitative skill."

That's been the experience in Victoria as well. As Daniel Atkinson, deputy fire chief for operations with the Victoria Fire Department, told me, "What we're seeing now is that because there is such a saturation of naloxone on the street and available to the end user, there's more self-administering or partner administering and less activation of first responders as a result of that, because I think it's being managed at the street level. Our guys arrive on site, and it would be another user who has already actually administered the naloxone on the street. They're so much better at it, we don't do it a ton. I guess these guys, they're pretty versed with the needle."

Unfortunately, not all jurisdictions that are in the midst of the opioid crisis have made naloxone widely and freely available. Shockingly, there are media reports that individual pharmacists who've taken the initiative to get naloxone out into affected communities have faced censure. A comprehensive review by the Canadian Pharmacists Association in November 2017 found that improvements must be made to increase access to naloxone across Canada. At the time of their review, only Alberta, Ontario, Quebec, Nova Scotia, the Northwest Territories, and

Yukon were providing free, unrestricted access to naloxone—and even then there were some barriers (e.g., in Ontario a valid health card had to be presented, which presents an impediment for some vulnerable populations). BC has since joined the list.

"Naloxone should be readily available to all Canadians at no cost, regardless of where they live," said the Canadian Pharmacists Association. "We therefore recommend that all provinces implement publicly-funded Take-Home Naloxone programs to ensure that naloxone is available to all residents without restrictions on eligibility, supply or cost. Furthermore, naloxone should be available through a variety of providers, including community pharmacies, community health centres, and first responders."

A recent death review panel by the BC Coroners Service recommended that everyone who's been released from incarceration and under corrections supervision in the community have access to a take-home naloxone kit, given how significantly overrepresented these individuals are in overdose death statistics. A program in the United Kingdom that gives prisoners these kits upon release was found to significantly reduce opioid overdose deaths among that population.

Remember Brandon Jansen? He was the 20-year-old who died of an illicit drug overdose at the Sunshine Coast Health Centre after being released from jail. I was shocked to read in the coroner's inquest that naloxone wasn't available at the recovery centre at the time he overdosed. The coroner's inquest jury recommended that all substance use treatment centres educate clients with opioid use disorder about the risks of relapse, ensure they understand about tolerance levels, provide training for staff on administering naloxone, and give patients a take-home naloxone kit when they're discharged.

——

Despite all the evidence that naloxone saves lives and that it's cost-effective and safe, I was surprised to find that some people are still opposed to making it widely available.

"Naloxone does not truly save lives, it merely extends them until the next overdose," said Paul LePage, Maine's Republican governor. In April 2016 he vetoed a bill to make naloxone available over-the-counter to people at risk of overdosing, or to their family members. It "serves only to perpetuate the cycle of addiction," LePage said.

That's like saying giving CPR to someone suffering a heart attack merely extends their life to their next heart attack. By LePage's logic, we should just let those people die too. Restricting access to a critical life-saving medication like naloxone is heartless and cruel. The research is clear: delaying the rapid distribution of take-home naloxone costs lives.

Likewise, an article recently made its way around the Internet claiming that naloxone encourages riskier drug use as a result of "risk compensation," the argument being that, given naloxone's availability, people will engage in riskier drug use because they perceive the chances of dying from an overdose as lower. The argument, along with the methodology behind the article, was thoroughly dismantled by numerous experts.

Indeed, researchers found that naloxone does not encourage increased drug use. To the contrary: there are studies showing the opposite. In one study, intravenous drug users who were educated and trained in how to respond to an overdose with CPR and naloxone saved the lives of their peers while decreasing their own drug use over a six-month period. Medical experts say that "this is likely because people who use opioids are very averse to naloxone induced opioid withdrawal, and opioid overdose education may reduce incremental risky behaviors."

Even Dr. Jerome Adams, the U.S. Surgeon General appointed by President Donald Trump, recently issued an advisory calling for naloxone to be made widely available to patients prescribed high doses of opioids, illicit drug users, people abusing prescription opioids, healthcare practitioners, family and friends of people with opioid use disorder, and community members. The simple message from Dr. Adams is this: "Be Prepared. Get Naloxone. Save a Life."

Another concern people might have about helping someone they believe is overdosing is that they could be sued if the person is injured or dies, even though they were just trying to help. But most provinces, including BC, have civil "good Samaritan" laws so that laypeople can't be sued for damages if they provide help during an emergency, unless they're grossly negligent.

Many public places now have automated external defibrillators (AEDs) to save the life of a heart attack victim when there's no time to wait for professional first responders. The same should be the case with naloxone. That means making naloxone, and people trained to use it, available at all venues where there's a chance of an overdose occurring. When UBC recently hosted a roundtable on the opioid crisis attended by people who use drugs (who sat at the table as experts alongside physicians and professors), it had several naloxone kits on hand for anyone to access. It wasn't promoting drug use—the medication was there for those who were already using or had in the past as a way to make sure they were safe.

Saving lives has to be our top priority.

"It was not a great leap for us to, for example, put naloxone in the hands of front-line police officers. They didn't need a lot of convincing," said Clayton Pecknold, assistant deputy minister and director of police services in BC. "That's not the case in Ontario, for example. The chiefs of police back in Ontario were resisting it. Surprising to me. Shocking to me, frankly."

———

"Addiction doesn't need to be a death sentence." It's a powerful declaration from PHS Community Services Society. And one aspect of that is educating the public in overcoming any reluctance to call for emergency aid.

Studies have found that bystanders often don't call 911 or seek medical help during a drug overdose because they're afraid of the police coming and the potential for criminal charges being laid. To reduce that barrier, on May 4, 2017, the federal Good Samaritan Drug Overdose Act became law in Canada. If someone experiences or witnesses an overdose and calls 911, this new law provides them with some limited legal protection: the police can't charge them with simple possession of illegal drugs, or for breaching conditions related to simple possession of illegal drugs (e.g., pre-trial release, probation orders, conditional sentences, or parole conditions).

"It's very recent. I mean, we saw these laws in the United States—I don't know how many dozens of States have a law like this—but in a lot of cases nobody knows about it," said Jordan Westfall, president of the Canadian Association of People Who Use Drugs. The police agree that many people, including some first responders, don't know about the law or are confused about how it applies. At least one senior official I met with in BC, who was responsible for overseeing training for front-line first responders in a major city, had never even heard of the federal Good Samaritan legislation. Research has shown that drug overdose Good Samaritan laws don't help much without effective education campaigns about their existence and scope. So there's much more work to be done to raise awareness about this new law.

There are also concerns that the federal Good Samaritan Drug Overdose Act is too narrow. "In theory," said a representative of Pivot Legal Society, "the principle behind the Act—to encourage calls to 911—is a good one, but if that actually is the goal, we feel that the way that the law is under this Act is inadequate. It provides actually quite minimal legal protections for people. It protects them [only] in instances of simple possession."

Indeed, the Act doesn't protect people from being arrested for offences other than simple possession, such as theft or possession for the purpose of trafficking—the latter a complex charge that involves a lot of police discretion and isn't well understood by people on the street. Nor does the Act cover those who've been charged with a criminal offence (other than simple possession) and are released on bail before their trial, or those who've been convicted and put on probation: these people will frequently have to respect a range of conditions (such as abstaining from drugs or alcohol). The Act doesn't provide any legal protection against charges for breaching those conditions or for outstanding arrest warrants (such as for missing a court appearance).

As Westfall told me, "I think they started with just simple possession, and I think it needs to include breach charges if people have outstanding warrants for non-violent acts. Those things would make people feel a lot more comfortable." Lawyers and healthcare advocates agreed that the legislation needs to be expanded to encourage people to call 911 during an overdose. "People who use drugs, particularly those who are street involved, still feel marginalized and vulnerable when they deal with police," pointed out Dr. Bonnie Henry, BC's chief medical officer.

There are also concerns about police attending non-fatal overdoses (where a person is experiencing an overdose but has not died) when all that's needed is medical intervention. If it's just a medical situation and no violence is taking place, there's arguably no public safety reason for the police to be there. And if people think police will come to a non-fatal overdose, that can deter them from calling 911 for help.

"People will not call 911 because they fear police attendance. It doesn't need to result in a charge. It's just a relationship of bad history with police—and it's fear of what could happen that oftentimes drives people into incredibly dangerous behaviour and cuts them off from the services that they need," said Pivot Legal Society. Police attendance at a non-fatal overdose could also be a problem for undocumented immigrants who fear deportation if they call 911—another issue that Good Samaritan laws often don't address.

"I think a lot of police departments throughout the country are still responding to non-fatal overdoses, and that's a deterrent for people to call 911, even with the Good Samaritan Act," conceded Inspector Spearn. "In Vancouver, we stopped going to non-fatal overdoses in 2006 as a policy. The only time we'll attend an overdose is if Fire or Ambulance request our presence for safety reasons, if it's an attempted suicide, and, of course, if it's an overdose death."

The VPD's approach made sense to me. The opioid epidemic is a public health emergency. Our criminal laws and criminal justice system have to get out of the way of first responders whose job it is to save lives and let people call 911 without fear. I was also convinced that we need to increase awareness of the Good Samaritan Drug Overdose Act and expand its legal protection to include immunity from prosecution for any non-violent offence and for related breaches of condition and warrants.

What's the whole point of our criminal law anyway? It's intended to save lives and protect people. We can't forget that.

———

Naloxone is a miracle drug that saves lives during an overdose emergency, but it's not a silver bullet for singlehandedly solving the opioid crisis. There are four reasons why.

First, giving someone who's overdosed an excessive quantity of naloxone puts them into withdrawal. And as we've seen, avoiding withdrawal is one of the primary drivers of opioid use by people with opioid use disorder. The naloxone that has saved their life can simultaneously compel them to quickly use again, even though they just about died. It may be hard to understand, but some people who are revived from an overdose can be angry because the naloxone has abruptly ended the pain-relieving effects of opioids that their body craves and that they've spent their scant money for. This need to stave off withdrawal symptoms, even at the risk of their own life, blatantly reinforces the fact that opioid use disorder is a relentless condition that effectively robs many users of their autonomy.

"It's one of the hardest things when we treat someone. In essence, you reverse their overdose with the naloxone, but they don't want to go anywhere," said Vancouver Fire Chief Reid. "They don't want to go to the hospital. It's exceptionally hard to have the same person overdose three times in a day and die on the fourth."

"That's happened?" I asked, finding it hard to believe.

"Yeah. And it's really frustrating," said Reid, referring to the strain on front-line firefighters who live the opioid crisis day in and day out. "They develop relationships, too. They have regulars."

Second, once someone has had a non-fatal overdose, they're at greater risk of overdosing again and dying. "I think a huge number of lives have been saved by take-home naloxone," said Dr. Evan Wood, executive director of the BC Centre on Substance Use. "Though that's resuscitating people in the moment. But if you don't offer other things, then obviously they remain at high risk of a subsequent fatal overdose. Actually, there's literature to show that individuals who have had a non-fatal overdose are at extremely high risk of subsequent fatal overdose."

Third, people may simply administer naloxone without other necessary medical interventions, such as rescue breathing. Unless an overdose victim receives sufficient oxygen to their brain during the time it takes naloxone to begin working, they can suffer permanent brain damage even if they're revived.

"Naloxone is unfortunately all too commonly considered just this panacea for the opioid crisis," said Staff Sergeant King. "In an acute situation, it should have been used together with rescue breathing and supportive CPR and all those other factors. Even our own police officers think, 'Oh, just administer naloxone and let it do its stuff.' People can suffer brain damage and other really terrible medical side effects."

As Dr. Bonnie Henry told me, "Opioids, artificial or natural, are respiratory depressants. People stop breathing, which is why we teach rescue breathing when we're teaching the use of naloxone. Until somebody comes back up with the naloxone, you want to make sure their brain is still getting oxygen. One of the biggest risks is an anoxic brain injury—brain tissues don't like being without oxygen and can die off very quickly. So there is a potential for permanent brain damage, depending on the individual. That can mean visual, that can mean cognitive, that can mean behavioural change and other changes as a result of that injury."

A senior health official in BC, who asked to remain anonymous, told me that there have been situations where patients can't get into an ICU in Vancouver because it's full of people who didn't quite get resuscitated or had too much brain damage due to overdosing.

While many medical experts I spoke to raised concerns about the long-term effects of repeated non-fatal overdoses, they noted that there has yet to be a definitive clinical study confirming the phenomenon. But social services providers and the courts are already seeing what they suspect is a link. "Every time the brain is deprived of oxygen, brain cells start to die," said Jennifer Breakspear. "We're starting to notice within our buildings and within the neighbourhood some folks who are deteriorating physically—with balance issues, with other issues, but also cognitively—and I raised this with the health authority."

"What we're seeing now are more and more people with signifi-cant cognitive impairment because they've got brain damage," said Judge Elisabeth Burgess with Vancouver's Downtown Community Court. "We've always had people with cognitive impairments and different kinds of organic brain damage: FASD [fetal alcohol spec-trum disorder], things like that, that aren't really treatable. They're not going to get better. They come through the court repeatedly. There's not much we can do for them. Sometimes housing and other healthcare will stabilize them a little bit and they'll commit fewer offences, but you can't really cure that kind of thing. We're adding to that population because of this overdose crisis that's happening."

Fourth, while take-home naloxone is saving lives, it's meant a recent notable decline in 911 calls and emergency rooms visits for overdoses. Everyone I spoke to was quick to point out that this is the result not of fewer overdoses but rather of an increasing number being dealt with by naloxone alone. BC's Take Home Naloxone pro-gram estimates that 911 was called in only about half of overdose events, even though it's the first and most important step in respond-ing to an overdose. One of the reasons to call 911 is that naloxone wears off in 20 to 90 minutes, after which an overdose can return.

"Not everyone wants to be in the emergency department," said Dr. Aamir Bharmal, medical health officer and medical director of communicable disease and harm reduction with Fraser Health. For example, about one-third of overdose patients leave St. Paul's Hospital in downtown Vancouver before they've been discharged. It's a lost opportunity to help them. "What we'd like to do is try to ensure that people who are overdosing obviously have as many opportunities and access points for treatment."

Naloxone is an essential life-saving medication during an overdose emergency. But if we want to keep people with opioid use disorder alive longer and have them get into treatment if and when they want to, a lot more is needed.

— 10 —

DON'T SUPERVISED INJECTION SITES ENABLE DRUG USE?

One has a moral responsibility to disobey unjust laws.
—*Martin Luther King, Jr.*

Sarah Blyth doesn't let rules get in the way of helping people. During the opioid crisis, it's rebels like her who've been challenging the status quo in order to save lives. I first heard about Blyth in the fall of 2016. She'd apparently set up a tent in a Downtown Eastside alleyway with a bucket of naloxone and was reviving people who were overdosing from fentanyl-contaminated street drugs. The media was calling it an unauthorized "pop-up" supervised injection site. I had to meet her.

After a few months of trying to pin down a time, we did finally meet one morning at Blyth's street-level office on East Hastings—the headquarters of the Overdose Prevention Society that she founded and leads as its executive director. We sat in a couple of mismatched chairs around a simple desk. She was wearing a light grey zipped-up hoodie and her hair was tied back with several wisps sneaking out. After she took a sip of coffee, she let out a yawn.

"I heard a bit from media stories, but I wanted to hear from you," I began. "How did you get started doing this?"

"Well, I worked for the Portland Hotel Society for 10 years," said Blyth. "In the very beginning of that I worked as a manager of a shelter called the New Fountain. It was created during the Olympics to get people off the street, into shelters." At the time, activists claimed that Vancouver was trying to brush the city's visible homeless population under the rug during the 2010 Winter Olympic Games. Sure enough, when the games were over and all the international visitors and media had left, they tried to shut the shelter down that summer. Blyth was having none of it. "We said no," she told me. "We kept it open."

That wouldn't be the last time she'd ignore officialdom in order to protect vulnerable people.

Blyth then started working part-time at Vancouver's Insite, North America's first "supervised consumption site." People can use their illicit drugs and obtain clean supplies, and they're monitored and helped if they overdose. Insite has an exemption from the federal minister of health, meaning that staff and clients are immune from criminal prosecution there, under the Controlled Drugs and Substances Act.

The Supreme Court of Canada overruled attempts by Prime Minister Stephen Harper's government to shut Insite down. Despite that ruling, Harper's government imposed a series of restrictions on applications for new supervised consumption sites. The process has since been streamlined somewhat by the federal Liberal government, but it's still lengthy and involved. When I first heard about Insite in Conservative circles, it was portrayed as a left-wing scheme that enabled illegal drug use and was open only by virtue of "judicial activism" by the Supreme Court. I had some doubts, but that's what I'd assumed as well. I remember people using words like "junkies" and "addicts"—words I used to use, too. I now know how hurtful and dehumanizing those labels are for people who use drugs.

"I also started working with the Street Market Society," Blyth continued. "I became the manager. It went from a market that was one day a week to seven days a week." The Society runs an open-air flea market on East Hastings Street. For $1 per table (if they can afford it) people sell clothing, electronic equipment, old video games and movies, personal hygiene products, and other small items. Most things look used, but some are probably new. The bazaar is closely watched by police.

"We started seeing a lot of overdoses in 2016 in the neighbour-hood," said Blyth. "I was trained because I worked at Insite. A few of us were trained but not everybody, so we started to get our staff trained. People were overdosing in the front and in the alley. And it was just happening so frequently that we decided to set up sort of an area in the back of the market, because it was mostly in the alley where the overdoses were. It was like a medic tent. We had needles, a place to get rid of needles, a bathroom, and volunteers watching to make sure nothing happened—because if you wait five minutes for an overdose to happen, then worse things are happening."

"What happens if there's an overdose?" I asked.

"They give oxygen with a machine, they give naloxone, they become experts in overdose prevention," said Blyth. "We get our training, some of it from paramedics, some of it from people who've been on the front line for 10 years at Insite."

Blyth and her group called themselves the Overdose Prevention Society. Their tent opened in October 2016 in the back alley between Pender and East Hastings streets, off Columbia. It looks just like any other alleyway in the area. There's garbage strewn about, people lying in sleeping bags on hard concrete, colourful graffiti-covered walls, grime covering the asphalt. Not the kind of place most Canadians are exposed to every day.

"We were busy all the time with people wanting our help," Blyth told me. "When people found out what was happening there was a bit of a political kerfuffle about whether we should be able to do that or not—because it's not a federally sanctioned thing, and we were on BC Housing property. And if we moved out to the city property, then they're in charge of what happens, and you can't have a tent there. There's all kinds of reasons why you can't have an injection site."

Blyth and her group were concerned citizens in a long-forgotten back alley. They were ignoring federal drug laws in order to save lives during a public health emergency that was happening right before their eyes. They'd heard an urgent cry for help, and they responded. It was an act of civil disobedience. It was an act of compassion and mercy.

"We just said, 'Well, we have to do it.' What is the alternative to doing that? It would be people dying," said Blyth matter-of-factly. "You can't really think about it too much, because if you start asking lawyers about legality, you start hearing a bunch of things you don't want to think about. And then you're probably less likely to do it, you know what I mean? I'm not a big fan of worrying. People are gonna die if you don't do something."

Three months after the overdose prevention tent opened, Vancouver Coastal Health gave the Overdose Prevention Society funding to keep going. Their staff includes "peers," people with lived experience using drugs who act as front-line responders helping fellow drug users. Some of the community workers in the Downtown Eastside are mothers who've lost children during the opioid epidemic.

"It took a little bit of time," Blyth explained, "but eventually everybody came around and said, 'Okay, well you can't really say no to people saving lives.' Actually, the police were supportive. They were one of the first to say, 'You know what, let them. There's no reason to stop them from doing it.' So that was good.

"The next move was the BC health minister said to the federal government, 'Can we sanction these?' And they said no. And the province did it anyways, which was pretty good on the part of the province at the time. They just said, 'You know what? You can say no, but we're going to do this because we know it's the right thing to do.'"

———

On December 9, 2016, BC Minister of Health Terry Lake signed an order authorizing overdose prevention services anywhere they'd be needed in the province during the public health emergency. "Overdose prevention sites" under Minister Lake's order are recognized by the province, although they're not exempt from federal drug laws as "supervised consumption sites" like Insite are.

When the Overdose Prevention Society got their authorization, they ramped up operations to try to meet demand. First they moved into a donated trailer on the same site, and then into a building right beside the street market where it had all started. They now have 24 booths for supervised consumption and an outdoor covered area where they can monitor people who are smoking their drugs. Vancouver Coastal Health evidently doesn't much like the smoking area—it violates anti-smoking bylaws. Again, Blyth isn't about to shut it down. These makeshift facilities are saving lives.

"How many overdoses have you reversed?" I asked Blyth. She handed me a report listing all the data. On average, there were 377 daily visits to the Overdose Prevention Society's site and 6.6 overdoses per week. By the end of 2017 the total number of visits had reached 175,284. There were 417 overdoses—all successfully reversed. Naloxone was administered to 397 people; 911 was called 153 times; and 70 people were transferred to the hospital. Some 90% of people who overdosed were revived before rescue services arrived. And there have been *zero* deaths.

Behind these remarkable statistics are real people whose lives have been saved. When I met some of the staff and many of the clients,

I was struck by how upbeat and friendly everyone was—that is, until Blyth mentioned that I was a lawyer. Then I got more cautious looks. I don't blame them. Blyth shared a couple of the comments she's received from clients and peers who work at the Overdose Prevention Society:

> I have personally overdosed and had my life saved at the Overdose Prevention Society. I have also lost over ten friends and family to overdose. I am extremely grateful for access to supervised consumption sites because a lot of us wouldn't be here today if it weren't for a place to use safely.
>
> —*Will, 26 years old*

> You guys have saved my life a few times and without the staff I wouldn't be here today. My parents would be planning my funeral instead of camping trips in the summer. There's frequently a lineup to get a booth and no one should ever be turned away from a safe place to use drugs.
>
> —*Taylor, 24 years old*

There are now at least 45 provincially recognized overdose prevention sites in BC, which together have had over 600,000 visits and reversed thousands of overdoses since Minister Lake's 2016 order. Some focus on serving particular groups, like women or Indigenous people.

"What we're finding is it's an avenue into helping people connect. And that's what saves lives," said Dr. Bonnie Henry. "They may get food. They may get somebody with a clean bandage to help them with their wound. They may get a clean pair of socks for the first time. They're not judged for their drug use, and so we think that these have turned out to be critical services for saving lives.

"From a legal perspective, Health Canada has said, 'Oh, well, okay. Maybe we'll give you temporary exemptions to run these sites.' And we're saying, 'No, no. They're not under the Controlled Drugs and Substances Act. They're medically necessary services under our own legislation and we don't want your exemption.' Because I don't want them to start thinking they can control whether we operate these or not."

"One of the other things we learned from the overdose prevention sites," a Pivot Legal Society representative told me, "is that there are groups of people who will access those sites because they're peer run and not overly clinical."

Sarah Blyth's off-the-grid overdose prevention site wasn't just some clickbait news story about a rebel with a cause. It's now part of a grassroots movement that's spreading across the country. In 2017, her team reversed an average of one overdose almost every day. If Blyth and others like her hadn't stepped in, the death toll would have been even greater.

———

What should our primary goal be in responding to the opioid crisis? To me, it's crystal clear: we have to save lives. That means dumping a century of discredited myths and stereotypes about substance use and being willing to consider all options. We need to use the best available evidence about the most effective medical treatments, public health interventions, and laws and policies to achieve that objective. So, what's the track record of supervised consumption sites?

"The thing you're seeing very clearly in our data is the fact that there hasn't been a single death at any supervised consumption or overdose prevention sites in the province. I think that speaks volumes," said Andy Watson with the BC Coroners Service. "It's crucial that people have somewhere where they can go where they know that they're going to be able to be helped if their drug supply is unsafe."

Supervised consumption sites literally have a perfect record in saving lives. There has yet to be a single documented fatal overdose at any of these facilities, anywhere in the world, *ever*. Since 2003, Insite has had more than 3.6 million visits from people injecting illicit drugs. Staff intervened to treat 6440 overdoses. Not a single person died.

"The purpose of supervised consumption is to ensure that people are safe," said Dwayne McDonald. "It's acknowledging that these people have an addiction issue and we want to make sure they're safe." Before the BC public health emergency was declared in 2016, Insite staff were seeing about one overdose per day. In 2017, that had risen to six overdoses every day, or 2151 people in total. Additionally, around that same time, Vancouver's overdose prevention sites reversed 1225 overdoses in their first year of operation.

When you consider the impact of supervised consumption sites and overdose prevention sites, it's an outstanding record. On average, in Vancouver one person died from an illicit drug overdose every day in 2017, while every day around ten survived an overdose at these sites. "Our position is that the science tells us, and the public policy tells us, that these sites work well in the midst of this acute crisis. They're a bandage to stop a chest wound," said Staff Sergeant Conor King with the Victoria Police Department. "When I look at the role of the police in the community, our single most important mission is to preserve life—and everything else comes after. If these things are preserving life, then they're the right thing to do."

How is it that no one has ever died at a supervised consumption site or overdose prevention site?

The answer is straightforward: they're places where those who have opioid use disorder can go to use those drugs instead of using alone. Someone is there to keep watch over them—and that person knows what to do if they overdose. These places provide life-saving emergency first aid to treat illicit drug overdoses. It's that simple.

By May 2018 Vancouver had seven supervised consumption sites and overdose prevention sites, all of them in the Downtown Eastside. Yet we know that overdose deaths are occurring throughout the city, province, country, and continent. These sites need to be dramatically scaled up wherever there are clusters of overdoses and overdose deaths occurring.

———

"Insite saves lives. Its benefits have been proven," wrote then-Chief Justice Beverley McLachlin for a unanimous Supreme Court in *Canada v. PHS Community Services Society*. The 2011 landmark decision ordered the federal government to grant Insite an exemption from federal drug laws. "There has been no discernible negative impact on the public safety and health objectives of Canada," found the chief justice.

More than 100 peer-reviewed studies of supervised consumption sites—30 of them specifically evaluating Insite—have appeared in top-tier medical journals. Many of the Insite studies were conducted by leading experts like Dr. Evan Wood, executive director of the BC Centre on Substance Use, and Dr. Mark Tyndall, executive director of the BC Centre for Disease Control. These studies found no evidence of negative impacts, but rather a host of benefits.

By providing clean supplies, supervised consumption sites can reduce the transmission of communicable diseases like HIV/AIDS and hepatitis C. A study in *The Lancet* found that after intravenous drug users started using Insite, they were 70% less likely to share syringes than users who didn't frequent the site. Supervised consumption sites also often provide other medical help to vulnerable populations, such as wound care and pregnancy tests. In 2017, Insite provided 3708 such clinical treatments to people who might otherwise never see a medical practitioner.

Another benefit of safe-use places is that they provide human contact that can be critical in helping people access treatment for problematic substance use. For example, Insite has an adjoining treatment facility called Onsite, which offers short-term beds and transitional housing along with addiction programs. In fiscal 2017–18, 433 clients went to Onsite and had an average stay of 11 days, while other clients were referred to different treatment services.

A study in the *New England Journal of Medicine* followed more than 1000 Insite users over a 15-month period. It found that "supervised injection facilities are unlikely to result in reduced use of addiction-treatment services," but instead people who regularly visited Insite were 1.7 times more likely to enroll in a treatment program than those who didn't come as often. Indeed, 18% of Insite users began a treatment program during the study period.

As Vancouver Fire Chief Darrell Reid told me, "I'm supportive. I mean they're going to inject anyways, so might as well be safe." Daniel Atkinson, Deputy Fire Chief for Operations with the Victoria Fire Department, echoed that sentiment: "On a personal level, I'm in favour of the safe injection site concept. I think it's invaluable. I think it saves lives and allows people an opportunity for care and treatment."

———

What about the impact of supervised consumption sites on the surrounding community?

"I think a lot of the benefit is that when people are using in these sites they're not using in the doorways and alleyways and corners and parks," said Staff Sergeant King. "So there's another ancillary benefit for the greater community."

A study published in the *Canadian Medical Association Journal* bears this out. It tracked public drug usage, including unsafe disposal of used syringes, in the neighbourhood surrounding Insite before and after it opened. Researchers found "significant reductions in public injection drug use, publicly discarded syringes and injection-related litter after the opening of the medically supervised safer injecting facility."

In another study, researchers looked at crime rates in the neighbourhood around Insite before and after it opened. They found no statistically significant change in rates of drug trafficking, assaults, or robberies. But there was a drop in vehicle thefts and break-ins (302 incidents pre-Insite vs. 227 incidents post-Insite).

The police see real value in Insite and regularly direct people there. A survey of 1090 randomly selected Insite clients found that 182 of them (17%) had been stopped by police while injecting in public and were told to go to Insite instead. Researchers saw this as doubly beneficial, concluding that "by referring people who inject drugs in public to Insite, police are helping to meet both public health and public order objectives."

Medical research has also found that supervised consumption sites reduce the burden on emergency services, such as ambulances and hospitals, by offering immediate support to overdose victims.

After looking at the mountain of evidence, I realized that during all my time in politics, including working as a senior advisor to a cabinet minister and the prime minister, I'd never seen a clearer case for a public policy intervention than there is for supervised consumption sites. These places are an essential life-saving medical intervention and a key part of responding to the opioid crisis. They keep people alive, and they offer them human contact that can be an entry point for treatment and other support. Yet despite all the evidence, and even as record numbers of people are overdosing and dying, in some North American jurisdictions strident opposition remains.

———

"I don't believe in safe-injection areas, as I call them," said Ontario's Progressive Conservative Premier Doug Ford on April 20, 2018, during the provincial election. "I'm dead against that."

A month earlier, Jason Kenney, leader of Alberta's United Conservative Party and current premier, had told the *Lethbridge Herald* that "helping addicts inject poison into their bodies is not a solution to the problem of addiction. I think the focus should be on interdiction and law enforcement to keep this stuff off the streets." The next day Kenney tweeted, "Why isn't the federal government massively increasing resources for the Canada Border Services Agency to interdict these poisons? Why isn't our federal government demanding that the Chinese government crack down on these factories?"

During the 2019 federal election, Conservative Party leader Andrew Scheer slammed the expansion of supervised injection sites as "terrible." There has been even more strident opposition to supervised injection sites south of the border. "SIFs [safe injection facilities] are counterproductive and dangerous as a matter of policy, and they would violate federal law," said the U.S. Attorney's Office for the District of Vermont. "As to policy, the proposed government-sanctioned sites would encourage and normalize heroin use, thereby increasing demand for opiates and, by extension, risk of overdose and overdose deaths."

None of these objections to supervised consumption sites hold any water. First, as we've seen, trying to crack down on the supply of illicit drugs has been futile, and has even backfired. It contributes to an increasingly toxic contaminated drug supply. The war on drugs has led to cheaper and more potent illicit narcotics. It hasn't worked to stamp out any other drug, and it especially won't work with potent synthetic opioids that can be manufactured anywhere in the world.

Not to mention those millions of letters and packages arriving every month from China, any one of which could contain fentanyl.

Second, as for preferring to get people into treatment rather than supporting supervised consumption sites, the two go hand in hand and are part of a more effective response to the opioid crisis. Supervised consumption sites keep drug users alive so that they can get into treatment when they're willing and able. As demonstrated by the *New England Journal of Medicine* study cited above, users of supervised consumption sites are actually more likely to enroll in treatment.

Third, the evidence shows that supervised consumption sites do not encourage or normalize drug use. A study in the *American Journal of Public Health* found that "the average Insite user had been injecting for 16 years. Only one person out of 1,065 reported performing their first injection at Insite. This strongly suggests that Insite has not promoted illicit drug injecting, but rather that it has attracted individuals with long histories of injection drug use." That's right, only one person was found to have had their first injection at Insite. Politicians might as well start blaming rap music for the opioid epidemic—that's how ridiculous their claims are opposing supervised consumption sites. As Leslie McBain, co-founder of Moms Stop the Harm, put it, "There was drug use when we didn't have safe consumption sites. All that's ever happened there is lives have been saved."

I was also impressed with the high level of support among law enforcement officers for safe consumption sites and the benefits they see in them.

"I personally have never met anybody who is a drug user who cites the availability of a safe consumption site as a reason why they use drugs," said Staff Sergeant King. "In my experience that hasn't been the case. I don't believe that they encourage drug use."

"In 22 years of policing, of drug enforcement, I can tell you pretty confidently that nobody became a drug addict because of Insite," agreed Inspector Bill Spearn with the Vancouver Police Department. "One of the big fears when Insite opened was that it was going to act as a big magnet, drawing in people who use drugs from all around the world to come to Vancouver. But the truth of the matter is that if you're an addicted person and if you live a few kilometres away from Insite, you're not going to go because you're just too sick to get there. People who use Insite live within a few blocks of it. It's not enabling. Really, it's just being humane with people. It's giving them clean supplies. Something as simple as clean water rather than using water from a puddle. It's a way of keeping people healthy and keeping them alive so that one day they can get into treatment."

Even the faith-based community organizations I spoke with were supportive of the important role played by supervised consumption sites. "I mean they help people. They reduce morbidity and mortality and so, for us, that's important," said Bill Mollard, president of Union Gospel Mission. Although his organization doesn't run any supervised consumption sites or overdose prevention sites, Mollard is convinced they play an important role. "Firstly, we're glad they do. If my daughter was in the Downtown Eastside, I'd be doing it personally every day."

I wanted to know what Sarah Blyth with the Overdose Prevention Society thought about politicians who oppose such sites.

"People will just die with no safe injection sites," she said. "We've saved hundreds of lives in the past year. That many people would be dead because of what they're saying. I would say, Don't vote for those guys, because they're idiots and they don't really understand the issue. And I think the public is gonna understand that they don't understand the issue because that will actually kill more people. Conservative people's children use opioids too. It's not a political issue, really; it's a health crisis issue, and there's things that can be done that are known and scientifically proven, legally proven, and economically proven about how safe injection sites help."

Politically motivated opposition to supervised consumption sites represents nothing short of playing politics with people's lives. It's driving a wedge based on fear and stigma to win votes. People are afraid of crime despite the fact that, according to Statistics Canada, police-reported crime has declined significantly since the early 1970s. But many voters can be easily manipulated to vote for so-called "tough on crime" measures that don't actually make them any safer. And by demonizing people who use drugs, there's political gain to be had by those willing to play that game. Even progressive politicians can get caught in the trap—delaying the expansion of supervised consumption sites in the face of local opposition that's based on nimby-ism and stigmatizing those who use drugs. And as a result of such delays, more people will die during the opioid crisis.

———

Vancouver has the most supervised consumption sites and overdose prevention sites of any city in North America. They're saving lives, yet they aren't enough. Record numbers of people still died. Although a further increase in safe-use places would undoubtedly help (they're all currently in the Downtown Eastside, as I mentioned above; many have limited hours; and sometimes there are lineups), new ideas are needed to reach people who are using and dying alone.

"What we need to be doing is looking at how we can make this a normal health service and provide it in a variety of different settings," said Dr. Paul Hasselback, a medical health officer with Island Health. "The overdose prevention sites serve a population within a range of about 500 or 800 metres."

"Overdose prevention sites, supervised consumption sites are great for a half-mile radius around them," agreed Jordan Westfall. "There's still people who just don't necessarily want to use them. I just think that it would be nice to get to the point where people didn't have to worry. But we do need this right now."

Some creative solutions are being launched so that people don't have to use alone. Peers are often first responders in the opioid crisis: these can be friends looking out for each other, or even strangers. For example, the Vancouver Area Network of Drug Users (VANDU) has a group of peers on foot doing overdose prevention in the Downtown Eastside, while PHS Community Services Society manages "Spikes on Bikes" teams that get around on bicycles with clean supplies and naloxone. There are major challenges in reaching rural and remote communities, and one way of addressing these are the mobile overdose prevention sites based out of vans operating in the BC Interior.

Another approach that's being used in social housing buildings when there's a spike in overdoses is "witnessed use rooms," where people who use drugs can go to use them under supervision instead of the much riskier alternative. "Individuals were in their own rooms and they were alone; they were injecting and overdosing and nobody would know," said Bonnie Wilson, operations director (Inner-City Eastside) and co–program lead for mental health and substance use at Vancouver Coastal Health. "We couldn't call it an overdose prevention site and we couldn't call it a supervised injection site, but what it would be is a designated space in a supported housing building where an individual could say 'I'm going to inject right now.' They would go in, they would inject, or they could come down there with a peer, a friend, another tenant in the building—it was a safe place for them to inject and have someone check in with them. If there was a concern, if there was an overdose, a staff member or the tenant could respond right away." Of course, these witnessed use rooms work only if the housing is low- or no-barrier, meaning that they won't kick you out for using illegal drugs. They know that people have mental health and substance use issues and they want to keep them safe instead of forcing them out onto the street to fend for themselves or silently die of an overdose alone in their room.

Fraser Health has even been working on some tech-enabled ideas to try to reach people, recognizing that there's no one-size-fits-all approach to overdose prevention. "We're in the process of developing something where somebody can use an app [that would] call in a response if they don't turn it off in a specific amount of time after using drugs," said Chris Buchner, director of communicable diseases and harm reduction at Fraser Health. "What is an overdose prevention site? It can be everything it needs to be."

These are all interesting ideas. But what came up again and again in my research interviews is that, despite the risk of dying, there's one big reason why people have continued to use alone during the opioid crisis.

"We haven't been able to deal with the stigma," said Linda Lupini, executive vice president of the BC Provincial Health Services Authority and BC Emergency Health Services. "The stigma is what's making people shoot up in the bathroom in their house and their parents don't even know they use drugs every day. Or the professional person, or the construction worker. Whoever it is. There's still this huge number of people who just won't tell anybody."

———

"Hey, I'm here to get my drugs tested."

"Folks will come in; they'll walk to the front counter," said Troy Balderson, downtown projects manager for Lookout Society, which runs the Powell Street Getaway in the Downtown Eastside. Balderson has a buzz cut, a goatee, and tattoos that travel along his arms and up his neck to just below his ear. He's also got a heart for people with addiction and substance use challenges.

"We'll bring them into the room. They'll sit with our technician. They'll pull out a very, very small sample. Put it on the spectrometer. He'll give them a breakdown," Balderson explained.

The Powell Street Getaway, which opened a supervised consumption site in July 2017 (almost nine months after its application was sent in to Health Canada), is one of just two locations in Vancouver that are piloting a sophisticated on-the-spot, no-questions-asked drug-checking program for people using street drugs. The Fourier-Transform Infrared Spectrometer (FTIR), shared with Insite, can detect a range of substances, including fentanyl. It can give detailed information about the composition of a sample in less than two minutes. Plus, it's portable. However, results can vary depending on what part of the drugs are sampled, since fentanyl may not be uniformly distributed.

The other way of testing for fentanyl is with test strips, which are being distributed to all supervised consumption sites and overdose prevention sites in BC. They're much cheaper, although after you mix your drugs in water and dip the strip into the solution, they offer only a basic yes/no indicator for the presence of fentanyl. So in order to know with more certainty whether your street drugs contained fentanyl and what else is in them, ideally you'd use both a spectrometer and a strip.

"I think drug checking is something that really should be rolled out in a huge way," said Dr. Evan Wood. "And despite announcements about drug checking, if someone wanted to go and get their drugs checked right now, I actually don't know where they would go to get that done." Indeed, unless it's during the very limited days and hours currently offered at Insite or the Powell Street Getaway, sophisticated drug testing isn't readily available for people wanting to know what they're actually getting from their dealer.

"Knowledge is power in these types of circumstances," said Dr. Aamir Bharmal, medical health officer and medical director of communicable diseases and harm reduction with Fraser Health. But although the medical experts, community organizations, and law enforcement officials I spoke to were supportive of drug checking, they also noted that it has its limitations.

What impact does drug checking actually have? Given the widespread contamination of the illicit drug supply, a positive test for fentanyl isn't much of a surprise anymore to people who regularly use such substances. There haven't yet been any published clinical trials on how it might directly affect substance use behaviours, so that's something that's being studied through Vancouver's spectrometer pilot. Preliminary data from Insite suggests that while regular opioid users don't tend to dispose of drugs that test positive for fentanyl, they're 10 times more likely to use less and 25% less likely to overdose. Drug checking is also seen as providing another opportunity to connect with illicit drug users. "What I've been hearing about the drug checking is the presence or absence of fentanyl. People haven't said 'I'm not going to use'; it's 'I might use a bit less' or 'I'll use safer' or something like that," said Dr. Bonnie Henry, BC's chief medical officer. "When they get that positive fentanyl outcome, they may be less likely to use alone—they'll use with a peer, or go to a supervised consumption site or overdose prevention site just to be sure there's someone there to help if they overdose."

Drug checking could also play a role in preventing casual or recreational drug users from overdosing, since they're typically not seeking fentanyl but rather other illicit drugs. For them, a positive fentanyl test could make a difference in their decision not to use that hit at all. "We'll do it for long weekends as well," Balderson told me. "Especially around the fireworks festival and stuff, we'll do extra testing. A lot of rave party drugs are going to come in—Ecstasy, suspected MDMA—you know, folks that go party on long weekends. If there's fentanyl in it, we've had people leave and say 'I don't want it.'"

I was surprised when I heard about another group of individuals who are using public drug-checking services: drug dealers. "Even the low-level dealers—some of them are my patients—who didn't realize that their own drugs had fentanyl in it," said Dr. Ronald Joe, medical director for substance use services at Vancouver Coastal Health. "In fact, they're the ones who actually came to Insite to check whether there was actually fentanyl in their drugs."

"They wanted to know if what they were selling had fentanyl in it?" I asked.

"That's right. It's fascinating," said Dr. Joe. "For the sake of themselves and also for the sake of the people—you know, the circle that they're actually distributing and selling drugs to. Because they didn't want to harm their small group."

Despite the apparent advantages of drug checking, bureaucrats have put up roadblocks by once again citing our federal drug laws—ones based on a prohibitionist model that is singularly obsessed with inanimate substances instead of living people. "Drug checking is another area where Health Canada actually said, 'Oh, no, you can't do that. It's in contravention of the trafficking provisions under the Controlled Drugs and Substances Act,'" said Dr. Henry. "So, how we got around that, people purchase their own drugs and they do the test. They don't actually hand a sample over to a technician. I think any changes that can make the drug-checking process easier would be helpful."

As a Pivot Legal Society representative told me, "There's a pharmacy I spoke with that was providing drug testing for folks who needed it with drug-testing strips, and they were actually issued a notice to stop doing so because it supposedly constituted trafficking.

The drugs were passing over, the doctor or pharmacist was testing and handing them back."

Some have raised concerns about how much reliance we should put on drug checking as a tool to respond to the opioid crisis. "All these tests—test strips, for example—aren't perfect," said Dr. Bharmal. "There's a little bit of a safety concern here in terms of thinking that if this is a negative test strip you have no concerns and you can just use these drugs with no repercussions."

Taking that even further, is it possible that drug checking could encourage drug use?

It turns out, no. A review of published research by the BC Centre on Substance Use found "no adverse effect on recreational drug using populations, refuting early arguments that these services may increase drug use in this population by offering a false sense of confidence."

"It's a piece of the puzzle that's important," said Jordan Westfall. "[But] I feel like we dedicate way too many resources to it right now. Honestly, most people, they don't have a choice. They know the drugs have fentanyl in them. You can't get that exchanged for other drugs.

"It's just way too much effort and money being put into that compared to just making sure people have a safe supply. It's counterproductive to ultimately a better drug policy. But we do need it right now. I'm sure there's people who rely on it too, but I just don't see the uptake of it that I think people were expecting."

I could see Westfall's point. While drug checking did seem like a good measure to help give both regular and occasional users information that can reduce the risk of overdosing and dying, the drug supply is still just as contaminated as ever.

11

IS PROVIDING "SAFE DRUGS" GIVING UP ON PEOPLE?

The lineup started to grow at 9:25 a.m. on Vancouver's Abbott Street at the corner of West Hastings. It was a sunny morning, the first of June, 2018. The doors to the Providence Healthcare Crosstown Clinic would open at 9:30 sharp, but only for five minutes before closing again for another half hour.

A middle-aged man walked out of the laundromat next door with a bucket of water and tossed it out onto the sidewalk. Another man strode by smiling, his boom box blasting "You Spin Me Round (Like a Record)," that 1985 hit by Dead or Alive. He walked past an elderly Indigenous woman wearing a red hoodie and lying slumped over on the sidewalk. A cane rested beside her. Her eyes were so puffed up she could barely open them.

A thirtysomething man arrived on his bicycle, locked it up, and joined the queue. His bright blue T-shirt read "Safe Drugs. End Prohibition. Expand Injectables." Then the doors swung open and a half dozen people slowly walked inside, the doors closing shut behind them. I went to the side entrance to meet Dr. Scott MacDonald.

The Crosstown Clinic was the first place in North America to offer prescription opioids in a supervised clinical setting to people with

long-term, severe opioid use disorder. The two medications it provides are used traditionally for pain relief: diacetylmorphine (also
known as "prescription heroin") and hydromorphone (also known as
Dilaudid). Along with the clinic's physicians and nurses are social
workers and counsellors to help clients with life-skills counselling and
housing referrals and connect them with legal assistance.

Years ago, when I first heard about giving prescription heroin to
people addicted to drugs, it sounded totally nuts. I assumed that it
was only enabling drug use and perpetuating the problem. But now,
in the midst of the opioid crisis, I knew I had to take a closer look at
the controversial program and examine the evidence for myself.

As thousands of people across the country die from using illegal
contaminated street drugs of unknown contents and potency, the
Crosstown Clinic provides legal pharmaceutical drugs of known contents and precise potency, dispensed and administered under medical
supervision to qualified patients. No one has ever died at Crosstown.

This type of approach has been used in Europe for years. So how
did the idea of providing those who are addicted to illicit opioids with
prescription opioids get started in Canada? Does it work? Should it be
expanded? And isn't giving someone drugs who's addicted simply
giving up on them?

———

In 2005, Dr. Martin Schechter from the UBC School of Population and
Public Health led the North American Opiate Medication Initiative
(NAOMI)—a randomized controlled trial (the gold standard of medical research) carried out in Vancouver and Montreal. Its focus was on
long-term, daily users of injection heroin who hadn't responded to
multiple treatment efforts and had been extensively involved in criminal activity—people whom society had basically given up on.

These individuals were randomly assigned to receive either oral methadone (the withdrawal management drug) or injectable diacetyl-morphine ("prescription heroin") up to three times per day under medical supervision. Both carry risks that need to be managed, so researchers monitored their use in the event of an overdose (which is a greater risk when people are using other substances).

The results of the NAOMI study were published in the *New England Journal of Medicine* in August 2009. It found that patients who received diacetylmorphine made greater improvement on all metrics than those receiving methadone, including their retention in the study, medical and psychiatric status, economic situation, and family and social relations.

"When people start on this kind of treatment they're using illicit opioids, injecting multiple times a day," explained Dr. MacDonald, physician lead at the Crosstown Clinic. We were sitting in one of the clinic's medical examination rooms, so I kept expecting him to check my blood pressure or something. Dr. MacDonald had short grey hair, black-rimmed glasses, and wore a long-sleeved checkered shirt with jeans. He spoke with the precision and calm of a clinical physician with decades of experience, but he was clearly passionate about help-ing his patients despite their seemingly insurmountable odds.

Since the NAOMI patients were being provided with known drugs under medical supervision, their lives were no longer dominated by the quest for contaminated street drugs and the often criminal or risky things they needed to do to get the money to pay for them. "People can instead focus on housing, their self-care, food. And ultimately we have had people go to school and work," said Dr. MacDonald. "We have a few people who have completed training programs at Vancouver Community College and other schools. People reconnect to families. We've had people who have had families and moved on, who are not on injectables anymore."

The NAOMI study also reported an impressive public safety benefit. Twelve months into the study, two-thirds (67%) of the patients who received diacetylmorphine had reduced their illicit drug use or other illegal activities, with an average reduction of illicit heroin use from 26.6 days a month to 5.3 and of monthly illicit drug expenditure from US$1200 to US$320. For those patients on methadone, illicit drug use or other illegal activities went down by 47.7%, illicit heroin use went from 27.4 days a month to 12.0, and monthly illicit drug expenditure went from US$1200 to US$400. In other words, patients using diacetylmorphine fared better on each of these metrics than those using methadone.

In short, NAOMI was a breakthrough study—the first to use prescription heroin as a means of treating severe, long-term opioid use disorder. But if the researchers and patients wanted to move the idea forward, they were in for a fight.

"We applied to Health Canada when people were leaving NAOMI to have continued access to diacetylmorphine, but Health Canada at that time said no," Dr. MacDonald told me. "So the study shut down. I think very many went back to the street and [its] associated consequences and risks. Many had found at last something that worked for them, and yet it was taken away."

———

With diacetylmorphine facing significant political and regulatory barriers in North America and elsewhere, researchers next set out to see whether hydromorphone—a more accessible prescription opioid pain relief medication—could also be beneficial for people with long-term, severe opioid use disorder who had failed multiple other treatments. That was the question posed by the Study to Assess Longer-term Opioid Medication Effectiveness (SALOME), which ran from 2011 to 2015.

Some 202 patients in Vancouver who qualified for the study randomly received either injectable diacetylmorphine or injectable hydromorphone up to three times a day under medical supervision for six months. They weren't told which medication they were receiving. They were also given access to physicians, nurses, addiction counsellors, and social workers. And they could choose to pursue other treatment options, such as methadone (to alleviate withdrawal symptoms) or detox. I asked Dr. MacDonald to tell me more about the patients enrolled in the SALOME study.

"Hepatitis C. Homelessness. Mental illness. Criminal involvement—80% of our folks had been in jail for at least a month. Some have been in jails for years," he said. "We selected folks who had an average 11 attempts at treatment and have been using for 15 years."

The findings from the SALOME study were published in the *Journal of the American Medical Association Psychiatry*. Interestingly, while most patients had initially said they'd prefer diacetylmorphine (prescription heroin), researchers found that most were unable to tell whether they were receiving it or the hydromorphone. Researchers also found that, overall, the two medications were equally effective in reducing illicit drug use. They concluded that when diacetylmorphine isn't available or hasn't been successful for a patient, hydromorphone could be an alternative. "If hydromorphone is all we have, it will work for a lot of people," Dr. MacDonald told me. "But here in Canada we've got access to both drugs."

Just as when NAOMI had ended a few years before, when SALOME wrapped up researchers tried to help maintain the treatment for those patients who were benefiting from it. The researchers had to ask Health Canada for special permission to keep offering each one diacetylmorphine under medical supervision. "We started sending in requests to access the Special Access Program [SAP] through Health Canada. There was a lot of back and forth," said Dr. MacDonald.

"Ultimately, at the end of September 2013, we got the first SAP approvals for diacetylmorphine. The same afternoon the minister of health at that time, Rona Ambrose, stood up in Toronto and held a news conference." That's when Ambrose announced she was intervening to halt the approvals, saying, "This decision is in direct opposition to the government's anti-drug policy. Our policy is to take heroin out of the hands of addicts, not to put it into their arms."

Even though SAP approvals had already been secured for some SALOME patients, the federal Conservative government quickly brought in regulations to prohibit physicians from prescribing diacetylmorphine. The Conservative Party even went so far as to send out a fundraising blitz to its members, with a spokesperson writing, "I was shocked to learn today that Health Canada approved applications to give heroin to addicts—against the wishes of our elected government. We're going to take steps to make sure this never happens again."

Just as when it had tried to shut down Insite, the Conservative government was again taken to court for trying to shut down an initiative that had proven to be not only safe and cost-effective but also reduced the risk of fatal overdose and actually reduced crime.

Larry Love was one of the SALOME patients who sued the federal government. While serving in the Canadian Armed Forces his knee had been injured, and he was honourably discharged in 1969. He moved to Vancouver and started using heroin to relieve his pain. Love even spent time in jail for activities related to his illicit drug use. He tried methadone but was unable to function on it. Love attempted detox over 50 times.

"It was a life of hell," he said.

Finally, during SALOME, his life stabilized. Love's doctor applied to Health Canada for Love's continued access to physician-supervised diacetylmorphine after the study ended, but was denied. Love returned to illicit heroin.

On May 29, 2014, Chief Justice Christopher Hinkson of the BC Supreme Court ruled against the federal government in the case. He held that physicians for Love and other SALOME patients should be able to continue to seek permission from Health Canada to provide supervised access and use of diacetylmorphine.

"We started getting SAP approvals again. It was funny. All these [approval] faxes used to come on a Friday before a long weekend," said Dr. MacDonald. "Ultimately the health authorities, pharmacare and the ministry, stepped up and said we can continue the program."

———

Today, the Crosstown Clinic has 150 patients who have long-term, severe opioid use disorder. About 80% of them receive diacetylmorphine and 20% receive hydromorphone; they inject it themselves, under medical supervision, at pre-set times every day. "They have seven minutes to inject and then we monitor them for 10 to 20 minutes afterwards. They're good to go at the end of a half hour or less, and the next group starts," said Dr. MacDonald. "People need to come two or three times a day for this to work. Most take a little bit of methadone or some long-acting morphine to sort of bridge them overnight."

In BC, owing to the opioid crisis, Health Canada recently added diacetylmorphine to its "List of Drugs for an Urgent Public Health Need." This means that physicians like Dr. MacDonald don't need to apply for special permission for every single patient they deem to require access to the drug. "We've been taking new patients since August," he told me. "We have a waitlist of over 300 people."

During the opioid crisis, access to injectable hydromorphone has started to slowly expand to some other clinics in BC. Not only are these interventions effective at saving lives, improving quality of life, and reducing illicit drug–related criminality, they're also cost-effective. A major study of the economic implications of these medications concluded that "[t]he costs saved through reduced involvement in violent and property related criminal activity and hospitalization outweigh the costs of both HDM [hydromorphone] and DAM [diacetylmorphine], and provide more benefit."

I asked Dr. MacDonald about the claim that providing prescription heroin to someone who's addicted is tantamount to giving up on them.

"Well, firstly, there's no recovery from a fatal overdose. That's painfully obvious," he said. "This needs to be managed just as a chronic manageable illness. And if somebody is coming here three times a day, and no longer having to engage in the illicit stream of opioids, they get housing, they may be working part time. It's a total success. What's the alternative? Using illicit opioids daily and being engaged in criminal activity just about every day. This treatment provides relief from that. It transforms people's lives and reduces the burden on taxpayers. If you're concerned about costs and crime, you need to expand injectable treatment options."

———

Dr. Schechter, who launched the NAOMI project that started it all, also points out that these programs don't just substitute illicit street drugs for drugs of known content and potency; they also provide other intervention opportunities as well: "It is the application of a 'bundle' of interventions that includes not only the provision of the pharmaceutical, but the opportunity for patients to benefit from up to thrice daily contact with doctors, nurses and counselors; the breaking of their cycle of criminality, sex work, jails, and hospitalizations; and the stabilization of their previously chaotic lives which made improved health outcomes extremely unlikely."

Dr. MacDonald concurs. "Opioid use disorder is a chronic manageable illness, just like diabetes or high blood pressure—and just like somebody with high blood pressure or hypertension, you've got first-line therapies that will work for most people. Sometimes people require more intensive treatment. If somebody had to take a blood pressure pill or a combination of blood pressure pills for 20 or 30 years or longer, would you question that? No. The management of opioid use disorder is exactly the same. The treatments we have—including injectable opioid agonist treatment with hydromorphone or diacetyl-morphine—we can show that when the other treatments haven't worked, this is better care."

In fact, European studies have found that the average length of diacetylmorphine treatment is three years. It's prescribed for opioid use disorder in the United Kingdom, Switzerland, Germany, Denmark, and the Netherlands.

"If this were any other disorder or medical condition or illness, do you think we'd still be in the position of this being the only place on the continent where you can access these medications?" I asked.

"Absolutely not," replied Dr. MacDonald.

"Why is that?"

"Stigma. Stigma against people who use injection opioids, stigma against injectable treatments, and stigma against prescription heroin."

———

"Get people access to clean drugs."

For Dr. Mark Tyndall, that's the simple answer to what needs to be done today to stop more people from dying during the opioid crisis.

Dr. Tyndall's demeanour is measured and professional, but his frustration is evident, and for good reason. With 20 years of clinical experience, he's now BC's deputy provincial health officer during a public health emergency—which means that not only is he the main public face of the province's response to the opioid crisis, but he also bears responsibility for coming up with innovative ideas. I recognized his angular face and straight brown hair from the times I'd seen him on TV talking about the issue.

Poster programs aimed at reducing stigma, housing and social services for users on the street, opioid summits, drug decriminalization—these are just a few of the ideas that have been proposed for dealing with the opioid crisis. However, for Dr. Tyndall, they're all too late to help those at risk of overdosing today. "We are really trying to focus the conversation back on how we address the poisoned drug supply," he explained. "Focusing on treatment as usual or other harm reduction as usual—it's just not going to cut it. As long as we're asking people every day to play Russian roulette with these drugs, people are going to continue to die."

The BC Centre for Disease Control is launching a pilot study in which a select number of people in Vancouver and Victoria at high risk of overdosing will receive hydromorphone pills two to three times a day at supervised consumption sites or supportive housing facilities. It's expected that participants will crush the pills and inject them rather than using contaminated street drugs. The pills are also substantially less expensive than the injectable form of the medication. "The idea," said Dr. Bonnie Henry, "is that you would transfer into this safe prescribed opioid instead of using toxic street drugs. Which is why we have some of the pilot projects that we're looking into really pushing some of the boundaries around provision of hydromorphone pills to people who are addicted—to enable them to use a safe supply rather than street drug supply."

Jordan Westfall, president of the Canadian Association of People Who Use Drugs, has a similar view. "We need to really just emphasize undercutting the street market as much as possible, and that means very low-barrier access points for people already using drugs to access safer drugs. You're interrupting the cycle of hustling that you have to do on the streets to be able to pay for drugs every day. That can mean sex work. That can mean panhandling. It can mean property crimes. All of that could be greatly reduced. It saves people; it saves our criminal justice system a lot of money."

Indeed, lawyers have noticed the impact when entrenched street-drug users are provided with pharmaceutical drugs instead. "I had a client whose record was unbelievable," said Mark Gervin, a criminal defence lawyer. "He was very violent. Nothing would get in the way of him and his drugs. The amount of horrible deeds that he left in his wake in his drive to get his drugs was incredible." Gervin estimated that this client was implicated in over 800 criminal incidents, all related to his illicit substance use.

"He had a host of problems, including a head injury, but I didn't see him for a while and I just assumed he was dead," Gervin continued. "All of a sudden he was arrested for break-and-enter or something. I went to see him. I'm like, 'Holy moly. Where have you been?' He says 'Well, I'm in the NAOMI project. They were giving me my heroin.' I'm like, 'What do you mean?' He said, 'Well, I didn't need to steal any-thing. I got my disability payments. I got my drugs. I didn't need noth-ing after that.' And then, of course, Harper came and cut it off, and then they ended up going to the Supreme Court, and then my client got it back. I haven't seen him now for a couple of years, 'cause he was back on the legal drugs. They were back supplying him."

Even the courts have taken notice when frequent offenders stop coming to court on new charges because they're no longer having to beg, cheat, steal, or sell their bodies for street drugs. "With opioid replacements, they're getting the high but without the danger," said Judge Elisabeth Burgess. "They're surviving longer and we're not seeing them as much. They're totally liberated now, they feel, because they show up at these clinics three times a day. They get their legal dosage and they can do other things."

The cost to the healthcare system of the ongoing crisis is another reason for looking at the provision of pharmaceutical opioids to those with opioid use disorder. "I'm supportive of anything we can do to stop telling people who are addicted that they have to buy what we know are toxic drugs," Linda Lupini told me. "We're all paying for and responding to this. So why are we not dealing with that on the front end? We're spending millions of dollars keeping them alive so they can keep going and buying toxic drugs. What I say sometimes to the Ministry of Health is, give them clean drugs."

Some of the strongest support I heard for dramatically scaling up a "safe supply" for those who use drugs was from the families who've lost loved ones during the opioid crisis. "A dead drug user will never recover. Our first step is to keep people alive," said Leslie McBain. "You can't force a person into recovery. It's dealing with what's real. There's always been drug addiction, there always will be drug addiction. We're not going to end drug use or addiction.

"Mitigating the crisis by providing people with safe drugs, if we do that, we'll still have addiction, we'll still have people needing to address their trauma, their pain, all those things, but they won't be dying, and they'll have a chance to recover. Giving up is the very opposite of what we're doing.

"Most people need medically assisted treatment. We've seen a change in that there are doctors who will prescribe Suboxone and methadone and diacetylmorphine, and these drugs that will help someone stay on track, and then taper down, and go into further treatment, which would include counselling and other supports. That's the way to go. We need to hugely increase capacity for those things. People can find those treatments and those options, but it's really hard."

Even the police are on board with the idea of substituting contaminated street drugs with medically provided opioids for illicit drug users. "If you were providing them with a clean alternative—something that they weren't going to die from and that was given under medical supervision that would allow them to stay alive long enough to get treatment—that would lower crime as well," said Inspector Bill Spearn. "Property crime. Things like theft from autos. You see a lot of drug-dependent sex trade workers. I mean, if they were provided with a clean opioid as an alternative to street drugs under medical supervision, then that wouldn't necessitate them selling their bodies in order to feed their addiction."

"Opioid assisted therapy programs that provide addicted persons with opioid medications must be made immediately and easily accessible in therapeutic and supported settings," said the Vancouver Police Department's 2017 report on the opioid crisis. "The goal of this recommendation is to give addicted persons a 'clean opioid' (with known contents) for their addiction and to prevent addicted persons from contributing to the organized and disorganized crime-fuelled drug market through purchasing and using contaminated street drugs."

But rolling out "clean" opioids or "safe supply" to those using illicit street drugs has to be done thoughtfully, cautions Dr. Evan Wood. "The main issue, and this isn't well understood, is that it has to be brought in in a way that prevents diversion; otherwise, you get more opioid-addicted people. This notion of 'Giving out opioids is the way to get out of this mess'—that's how we got into this mess. So more of that is not going to get us out."

In order to treat people with opioid use disorder, Dr. Wood wants to see witnessed injection, evidence-based recovery services, and the ability to obtain prescription opioids from a pharmacy or clinic (along with strategies to prevent people from selling what they've obtained). His organization has released a report that also calls for the creation of "heroin compassion clubs" so that those who use drugs could legally source a safe supply that they could purchase. But he cautions that providing access to a safe supply isn't all that's needed.

"Giving somebody the clean drug is better than the alternative," said Dr. Wood, "but just giving them the drug doesn't solve the rest of the issue."

− 12 −

HOW CAN WE HELP
PEOPLE STOP USING?

At 19 years old, Jordan Miller realized that he had a problem. He went to his mom, Leslie McBain, asking for help.

"We used to say Jordan was over-partying when he was a teenager," said McBain. "He was drinking with his friends, smoking pot. It seemed to increase over ages 15 to 19, and became a problem specifically with alcohol and cocaine. We got him into rehab. He liked it there. I mean, he did well. He came out and was good for a little while, and then he just started up again."

Miller had launched his own small business installing wood stoves and chimneys in the Gulf Islands along the southern coast of British Columbia. But he had a back injury on the job and went to his family doctor to get help.

"That doctor gave him oxycodone," said McBain. "He gave it to him in ever-increasing amounts over about seven months—even after I'd gone to the doctor, who's also my doctor, saying don't give this kid opioids, he's at risk. He thanked me for the information and continued to do that.

"Jordan went to him and said, 'I'm addicted, I need help.' The doctor grew angry and basically fired him as a patient. There was no offer of support or treatment or anything like that."

Left to fend for themselves, McBain helped her son get into detox again for a 12-day stint. She tried unsuccessfully to find a doctor who could prescribe Suboxone—a medication to help treat opioid use disorder by reducing the symptoms of withdrawal and reducing cravings. She also looked for a psychiatrist with experience in helping people like Jordan, but wasn't able to find anyone.

McBain's desperate attempts to get help from professionals with the necessary expertise are not unusual. Many of the substance use disorder experts I spoke with highlighted the urgent need for up-to-date training for healthcare professionals to meet the needs of patients during the opioid crisis.

About four or five months after leaving detox, Miller relapsed and started taking drugs again. "What he did was, he doctor shopped. He went to about five different walk-in clinics," said McBain. "He was very charming and looked like a person legitimately in pain, and was able to get hydromorphone, Xanax, Citalopram, just a little array of drugs. It certainly helped him from going into withdrawal. One day he just took the wrong combination of those prescription drugs and it stopped his heart. He was alone in his apartment in Victoria and his girlfriend found him."

Miller died on February 4, 2014, at the age of 25.

"It's the worst tragedy that can befall a parent, certainly, and the family. It ripples outwards in its impacts," said McBain slowly. "He had a girlfriend, he had an apartment, a dog and a cat, he had his business, he was sort of setting out on his adult life. It can happen to anyone."

McBain filed a complaint with the BC College of Physicians and Surgeons against her son's family doctor. Soon after Jordan's death she spoke to Dr. Evan Wood, who encouraged her, when she was ready, to consider becoming an advocate for families like hers.

"I met two women who are both from Edmonton who had also lost sons to drug harms, and the three of us decided to start Moms

Stop the Harm," said McBain. "I think the first thing we did was create a Facebook page, and we've grown in the last three years from three of us to almost 500 people now, families across Canada, sadly. We provide support for families who are grieving; we try to support people who have loved ones in active addiction."

Moms Stop the Harm also advocates for a more compassionate drug policy. It now has chapters in every province, and is regularly consulted by various levels of government. McBain has also become the family engagement lead at the BC Centre on Substance Use, meaning she helps ensure that the organization's work is informed by the experiences of families who've been affected by the opioid crisis. It was at their office in downtown Vancouver where I met with her.

"The people who have lost a child—we see a person who's immobilized in grief in the first months," she told me. "They get numb, they go into deep, deep grief. They're not able to work, they're hardly able to often communicate with family. They find that people have a lot of stigmatized thinking around drug deaths. There's a difference if a kid dies of cancer. There's a different kind of reaction from family members and people around them to when a child dies of a drug overdose."

Since her son passed away, McBain has learned a lot more about opioid use disorder and what families can do to help loved ones in active addiction. "We tell them first of all to take care of themselves," she said. Then, when it comes to those who are addicted: "Love them. You want them to just get the heck out of there, get out of my face, go away, do your thing somewhere else. Most families don't know very much about addiction. I was the same. Check out what's in your community for treatment; see what kind of physicians you can find who will treat—because the first line is your family physician, and if your family physician has a clue about addiction and how to proceed, you're on a good path. Often that hasn't been the case, so that's why we really promote doctor training, medical professional training in substance use disorder.

"The people who have loved ones in active addiction, they have their challenges and they sometimes can't navigate their way into the system because, as Evan Wood always says, we don't have a system— it's fractured and we need to build one. We try to help them navigate so that they can get the support they need to stay well and help out their loved one," McBain told me.

"As I often say, if I only knew then what I know now, I'd like to think I could have saved my son."

———

When most people think of substance use treatment, they think of detox—going cold turkey, abstaining altogether. The idea is that if someone is going to stop using a substance, they should just stop using it entirely. Indeed, that's the dominant model most people have in mind when dealing with substances like alcohol. However, the problem is that applying such an approach to opioid use disorder can have deadly consequences.

"We've seen for a number of folks that getting off opioids isn't the same as getting off alcohol or some other things," said Jennifer Breakspear. "Going off cold turkey and being abstinent and then relapsing—there are much greater risks of overdose and death."

Yet many treatment and recovery centres for people addicted to opioids are still based on an abstinence model. That was the case with Brandon Jansen (in Chapter 7) and Jordan Miller (at the start of this chapter), both of whom tragically died from opioid overdose—one while in detox and the other shortly after leaving it. What do leading medical experts have to say about abstinence-based treatment?

"People who go to detox from opiates and then go back into their community lose their tolerance very, very quickly," said Dr. Bonnie Henry. "So the probability of relapsing and dying the next time you use goes up dramatically. We've seen quite a lot and you've heard stories in the news about people who have been in recovery, and then they relapse and they die."

"We know that with leaving an abstinence-based rehab program, the relative risk for a fatal overdose goes up," Dr. Paul Hasselback told me. "So it's not something that's been recommended." After we spoke he sent me a study published in the *British Medical Journal* which found that "patients who 'successfully' completed inpatient detoxification were *more* likely than other patients to have died within a year." I had to read that again. People who'd managed to finish their intensive detox program were more likely to die from a drug overdose than those who failed to complete the 28-day abstinence program. This so-called "treatment" was actually making things worse.

As a result, new medical guidelines on treating opioid use disorder strongly recommend against detoxification alone, since "this approach has been associated with elevated risk of HIV and hepatitis C transmission, elevated rates of overdose deaths in comparison to providing no treatment, and nearly universal relapse when implemented without plans for transition to long-term evidence-based addiction treatment."

There are also major concerns that residential treatment and recovery facilities can vary widely in quality. "Right now, recovery homes, for example, are unregulated, and they can do anything they want," said Dr. Henry, speaking about the situation in BC. "There's no programs. There's no standards. And they get money from the province—and some of them maybe have good results, some of them maybe not."

"In fact," Surrey RCMP Inspector Shawna Baher told me, "there's several houses that are basically, truth be known, crack houses, but they're using the term 'recovery home' in an effort to try and run a flop house or a boarding house."

What's heartbreaking is that families desperate to help their loved ones can end up paying exorbitant fees for so-called treatment and recovery programs that aren't based on any scientific evidence and aren't accountable for their outcomes. I was surprised to find that there are no clinical trials or meta-analyses showing residential treatment to be effective. In fact, relapse rates are 60% to 90%. Yet residential detox programs are often the first thing people think of when they learn that a loved one is addicted to illicit drugs. On top of that, these private programs can be incredibly expensive. "I've seen them cost $35,000 a month," said McBain. "How are people affording it? Only the people who can afford it, afford it. And that tells you a lot right there. A lot of these recovery centres that are so expensive do have a certain number of beds for people who don't have the money. There's some sliding scale, but I don't think these really expensive recovery centres have any more success. I've heard of people remortgaging their homes, using all their retirement savings, things that they never expected to have to do in their life plans. That's just such a tragedy given that a lot of the centres don't have great success rates."

I'd do anything in my power to save my own child's life. How could you not? So it's all the more upsetting to think of those vulnerable families who've spent their life savings on detox programs—programs that were not only ineffective but put their loved ones at greater risk of fatal overdose during relapse. And even if abstinence-based treatment does play a role for a limited number of people, organizations that operate in this way without informing patients of the risk raise big ethical and legal issues.

Politicians have often said we need more "detox beds," and that if people could "just stop" using, we'd reach a solution to the crisis. If only. We know that's not how it works.

So what's really needed to help people with opioid use disorder?

———

Two hours.

According to medical experts, if someone who's addicted to opioids asks for help, that's the optimal time you've got to get them into treatment—an all-too brief window before the pull of their addiction once more overwhelms their will to escape it.

"If you knew someone who was addicted to illicit opioids and they asked for help in getting into treatment, where would you go?" I asked.

"I wouldn't have the first idea where to start."

That's the answer I got from Bonnie Wilson, co–program lead for mental health and substance use at Vancouver Coastal Health. And if *she* didn't know where to go for help—in the very city hit hardest by the opioid crisis and in a country where finding treatment in rural areas is even more challenging—what chance would others have? Later, as I continued my investigation, I would find out.

"We've never had a proper addiction care system in North America, maybe worldwide. We don't have a system of care here like people with other illnesses enjoy and can access," said Marshall Smith, senior advisor for recovery initiatives for the British Columbia Centre on Substance Use and chair of the British Columbia Recovery Council. "We got here because we didn't give a shit about people with substance use disorders."

"A lot of money, a lot of resources initially went to harm reduction initiatives and very little went into treatment," said Inspector Bill Spearn. "Almost four years into the crisis we're finally just starting to see some of the treatment options come online, but it's not proportionate to the problem. People who use drugs and are addicted to drugs have a medical problem and, really, throwing them in jail is not going to solve this problem."

According to a 2017 Vancouver Police Department report on the opioid crisis, "Research has provided evidence-based options for treatment that reduce overdose deaths, reduce the negative impacts on communities, and reduce costs." Its chief recommendation was to provide "treatment on demand" for people with opioid use disorder. Interestingly, the police force didn't recommend stricter laws or more money for enforcement. Instead, they wrote, "we must invest in creating effective addiction treatment and realize the widespread public safety and public health benefits that would result." Even the police are saying that the answer isn't more law enforcement, it's greater compassion.

———

New national guidelines for treating opioid use disorder were published in the *Canadian Medical Association Journal* in March 2018. They broke ground, in the midst of the opioid crisis, by strongly recommending "opioid agonist treatment" as a first-line treatment, specifically the use of a prescription medication called Suboxone. Suboxone, which comes in pill form, is a combination of buprenorphine (a partial opioid agonist that prevents opioid withdrawal and cravings) and naloxone (which reverses the effects of opioids, as we saw in Chapter 9). I asked Dr. Mark Tyndall how Suboxone works.

"For the person who says 'I'm going back to school' or 'I've got a job' or 'I need to be straight,' Suboxone is a great drug," he told me. "You won't get high from it, but it will stop you from withdrawing, and we can stabilize you. And there's good literature to suggest that for a lot of people that's very effective. But there's also good literature to suggest that, if you're not ready for it, then it won't work for you. Many people—and I'd actually say most people who are on these programs—are on and off them. It's just the way addiction goes."

By preventing withdrawal and reducing the cravings, Suboxone can help regular users stop using contaminated street drugs or misusing prescription opioids. They can get further supports, like individual or group counselling or residential care.

"I'm a huge fan of Suboxone," said Marshall Smith, who is himself in recovery from addiction. "I think of Suboxone like a scalpel: in the hands of a trained surgeon, it's a life-saving instrument. We use Suboxone all throughout our treatment centres and in the recovery homes that I directly supervise. I've seen phenomenal outcomes."

Suboxone is now available in BC through prescription from any physician and is covered by pharmacare, which isn't the case in all jurisdictions. Many doctors are still learning about it, so their training and education is crucial in ensuring that this first-line treatment is made widely available.

Fortunately, Rapid Access Addiction Clinics have begun springing up in cities like Vancouver and Victoria. These clinics, I discovered, are the places to go during that two-hour window after someone with opioid use disorder asks for help. Depending on the clinic, people can either walk in on their own or get referred by doctors, nurses, or social workers. The clinics provide evidence-based treatments like Suboxone or methadone on a short-term basis to help stabilize patients before transferring them to a healthcare provider in the community. Importantly, a health card isn't needed to access these services, and they're free.

Compared with more traditional and well-known opioid agonists like methadone, Suboxone is considered a better option overall for most people with opioid use disorder. Those being treated with

Suboxone have a significantly lower risk of fatal overdose than those on methadone, both during and after treatment. As well, Suboxone has fewer and less serious side effects; it's easier to take on an ongoing basis because once the person has stabilized they can get a prescription to take it at home; and there's no concern about its being diverted to the illicit market since it doesn't provide the effects people seeking illicit drugs desire.

"The other secret is that a lot of people who are on methadone continue to use illicit drugs," explained Dr. Tyndall. "A methadone patient can take a day off and say 'I got some money today. I'd rather use heroin. I'm not going to pick up my methadone.' And their methadone would have worn off, and they get to use heroin for the day. Suboxone doesn't work that way. It sticks around more."

But Suboxone isn't a magic pill to make everything better. It doesn't make the underlying reasons for someone's addiction go away. Instead, they can come back fiercely to the surface.

"They feel very normal on Suboxone. The discussions I've had with people, they feel *too* normal," said Dr. Tyndall. "Like you have nothing. You've blown all your relationships. You live in a shabby SRO [single room occupancy] somewhere with cockroaches on the wall, and now you're not high anymore and you're not withdrawing. You're just bored and irritated and all the trauma that you started drugs for starts coming back again. If the options I give them are Suboxone or nothing, when I know they're going to buy fentanyl and any one of those times they could die, I think we have to do better than that."

There are other important limitations of Suboxone. For one, it can be extremely dangerous to use Suboxone with alcohol or other drugs like benzodiazepines (medications such as Ativan, Xanax, or Valium). So someone who has opioid use disorder and other substance use issues may not be able to use it at all. And although Suboxone and methadone can be helpful in stabilizing people, it can be difficult to effectively taper off these medications. Most attempts to taper down are unsuccessful. Still, researchers believe that "there are increased odds of success when doses are reduced gradually with longer periods of stabilization." As Bonnie Wilson told me, "There are individuals who are wanting to get off opioid agonist therapy. Get off the methadone, get off the Suboxone. We haven't done enough with the rest of our system to really support that."

While it was encouraging to hear that Suboxone is effective at helping some people stop using illicit street drugs and reduce their risk of a fatal overdose, Dr. Tyndall had raised serious concerns about its efficacy for many entrenched illicit drug users. These first-line treatments just aren't effective for approximately 10% of people with opioid use disorder. And more than half of those who start treatment with Suboxone or methadone discontinue it in the first year and relapse. Many are unwilling or unable to stop the self-medicating effects from opioids. That's where "safe drugs" again come in: they can help reduce the risk of fatal overdose.

———

Medical experts say that with the right treatment and follow-up, people with opioid use disorder can have sustained long-term remission. Some can benefit from moving between the evidence-based treatments described in this chapter (such as medications like Suboxone and methadone to reduce cravings and withdrawal symptoms so that they can use less drugs or abstain altogether) and those mentioned in the preceding chapter (such as opioid medications like diacetylmorphine and hydromorphone to help them stop or reduce their use of contaminated street drugs). The new guidelines for opioid use disorder say that residential treatment and psychosocial treatment (such as cognitive behavioural therapy and contingency management) may help some people and can be one part of a long-term addiction management approach, although they also note that there isn't strong evidence in that regard. In short, there's no one-size-fits-all approach. Treatment has to be patient-centred and responsive to individual needs. After all, every person in long-term recovery has their own unique story.

Controversially, a significant majority of Canadians recently polled want people who use illicit drugs to be forced into treatment against their will. But government- or court-compelled treatment for people with opioid use disorder is a horrible idea. "I don't think we have any good evidence that court-ordered treatment management, rehab, therapies of that nature have a role to play in long-term sustainability," said Dr. Paul Hasselback. "We've seen that in the past. We know it doesn't work for alcohol-related dependency. There's no reason to believe it's going to work here, and the interventions are not long enough to actually be sustainable." And as Dr. Ronald Joe told me, "Other jurisdictions have tried involuntary treatment. It doesn't work very well. In China, for instance, they've actually since changed it from an involuntary to a voluntary system now as a result of the fact that it didn't work. Most jurisdictions in the world would have a paradigm that addictions treatment is voluntary. A person voluntarily takes it on versus being forced to take it."

And when it's on a voluntary basis, the long-term benefits of treatment can be significant, not just for the individual, but also for their family and for society as a whole. The U.S. National Institute of Drug Abuse estimates that every $1 spent on addiction treatment saves the healthcare and criminal justice systems up to $12. Try getting that kind of return on the stock market.

Other assistance may be needed for those trying to recover from opioid use disorder, such as housing and employment support. Yet it's often family members who are left to advocate for their loved ones to get them the help they need. "I know a mom in Victoria whose daughter wanted to die because she was so addicted—she couldn't get the drugs and she'd get sick and all these terrible things," said Leslie McBain. "That mom, who's now one of our leader moms, pushed for about a year and a half to get her daughter the treatment she needed, the housing she needed, the counselling she needed. But the slog—navigating that for her was a full-time job. That would never happen with any other disease. It wouldn't."

———

One critique I've heard about the medicalized model of addiction treatment is that it doesn't address the underlying reasons why someone has opioid use disorder—reasons that we now understand to be a combination of genetic and "environmental factors," such as trauma.

But one organization that's championing a greater recognition and role for wellness in helping people with opioid use disorder is the First Nations Health Authority. As Dr. Shannon McDonald, its acting chief medical officer, told me, "Everything we do at the First Nations Health Authority is done with a holistic perspective. We are always looking at people's physical health but also their mental, spiritual, and emotional health within the context of their particular environment. When we deal with anybody, especially in mental wellness and substance use, we always have to look at it in the context of their whole life. We often talk about not having a drug problem in our community, but as having a pain problem," said McDonald. "Sometimes it's physical pain. It could be individual trauma, something in their life that they're struggling to cope with. It could be family, community, nation, historical trauma. All of those things contribute to an individual's relationships with opioids or other substances as they move forward.

"[With] people who've had severely traumatized lives, to just turn around tomorrow and say 'Here. Take pill X instead of substance Y' without dealing with the underlying issues of poverty and racism and trauma, we're never going to get any closer to a solution."

I could see Dr. McDonald's point. I'd heard a related concern expressed by Marshall Smith.

"I think that we're in the midst of an addiction crisis, and I know that a lot of people like to focus on the actual drug itself," he said. "No matter what the substance is that people are using out there, this is a people problem. This is a crisis of community. It's a crisis of connection. It's occurring in people and in their lives, and so through my viewpoint the solution lies in people, not in drugs, and other processes."

While first-line opioid agonist treatments like Suboxone or methadone can help stabilize people with opioid use disorder, and providing a "safe supply" of clean drugs like diacetylmorphine or hydromorphone can help keep them alive and reduce criminality and health risks, there's also a need for a long-term response that helps people in a more holistic way. Although our immediate objective during this crisis must be saving lives, our long-term goal should be helping people deal with the underlying pain, trauma, and other reasons that either caused them to begin using illicit drugs in the first place or are barriers to their sustaining recovery so that they can live full lives, free of the enslavement of substances. And that will take a major societal effort—one that Indigenous communities that have been hardest hit want to see become a reality.

In addition to recommended medical treatments, the holistic approach championed by the First Nations Health Authority for Indigenous people involves making culturally based treatment options available. That includes access to counselling, engagement with Elders, and traditional practices to support those with substance use disorders on their healing journey. "On the land" treatment is an innovative approach being used in Indigenous communities across Canada to help people get respite from often hectic, chaotic lives that can be consumed by substance use. Participants live on the land together and are provided with emotional, mental, and spiritual support. They engage in traditional practices and cultural activities. This helps restore and strengthen connections to their culture and identity that have been horribly damaged by colonization as well as racism and discrimination against Indigenous people. It's also an opportunity to develop deep, long-standing relationships with fellow participants, Elders, and facilitators.

There's also a recognized need for a holistic response to the underlying causes of their addiction and the obstacles to their recovery, among them homelessness, unemployment, and mental health issues. Many people I interviewed spoke of the need for "wraparound" services—not only medical care based on the latest research but also support with such related needs as housing, vocational training, and counselling. That would constitute a much better and more cost-effective approach than how we deal with these social issues today, which is to silo them off and ignore the obvious interconnections between them.

"Allowing people the dignity of a home, potential for employment, support services to deal with their trauma as well as medical services to deal with substance use is going to take us a lot further than putting people in jail for short periods of time," said Dr. McDonald. Unfortunately, instead of addressing the underlying challenges people are facing in their lives, our abiding societal response to illicit substance use has been just that—to punish people who use illicit drugs and brand them as criminals.

— 13 —

WON'T DECRIMINALIZATION
MAKE THINGS WORSE?

I never once saw Jim smile. When I met him he was in his late forties—twice my age at the time. He was unemployed, just trying to get by in downtown Toronto. He had grey, dishevelled hair and his clothes were well-worn and dated. One day a police officer stopped Jim and asked him for his identification (that's never happened to me and probably never will—white professionals like me don't get carded).

Jim riffled through his pockets and out dropped a little piece of plastic wrap. The officer picked it up. It contained a small amount of crack cocaine. Jim was charged with illicit drug possession.

When I was a second-year law student at the University of Toronto, Jim was one of my first clients at the Downtown Legal Services clinic. I had one shoplifting case under my belt and an assault trial scheduled in a few months. Another client had paranoid schizophrenia and was facing stalking charges. The work at the clinic was exhilarating, terrifying, and humbling all at the same time. We were trying to help people who were in trouble with the law but couldn't afford a lawyer or get legal aid. On days when I had court appearances I'd wear a suit to school just to try to look the part.

My first step was to read through the offence to see what the Crown prosecutor had to prove and find out how much hot water Jim could be in if he was found guilty. The Controlled Drugs and Substances Act is federal legislation that makes it a criminal offence to possess illicit drugs such as heroin, cocaine, methamphetamine, and fentanyl. A first-time offender with a small amount faces a maximum fine of $1000 and up to six months in jail. That doubles for a subsequent offence. If the Crown prosecutor decides it's a more serious situation, they can indict the accused; the law provides for a maximum penalty of seven years' imprisonment. There are separate offences for trafficking and possession for the purpose of trafficking, both of which have a maximum penalty of life imprisonment.

In first-time drug possession cases like Jim's, Crown prosecutors seemed to want people to plead guilty and pay a fine: a quick and easy resolution for the prosecutor. But for the accused it meant a criminal record that prevented travel outside of Canada and made it even harder to get a job. And for the impoverished clients who qualified for our legal clinic, paying a fine was out of the question. It didn't offer them any support, and it wasn't going to do anything to stop them from using again. It just punished them and set them up for even more legal troubles—kicking them when they were already down. In retrospect, the entire process seemed less than pointless.

Fortunately for Jim, owing to mistakes the police had made he was able to avoid both a fine and a record. From a legal perspective it was a win, but for him it just meant that this time he'd be left alone. I never heard from Jim again. I wonder what happened to him.

———

When I started researching the opioid crisis, I promised myself to keep an open mind. It was already clear to me that the status quo had been unable to stem the tide of illicit drug overdose deaths. And I knew that one of the most controversial and challenging issues I'd eventually have to tackle was whether we should decriminalize illicit drugs—making it no longer an offence to possess them but still a crime to manufacture, import, or traffic in them.

Now, as I stepped back and looked at everything I'd learned and experienced over the past few months, it became clear that our current prohibitionist approach, rather than lessening the opioid crisis, is actually exacerbating it. It's having a devastating impact on people who use illicit drugs, most notably on regular users who have opioid use disorder but also on those who use drugs occasionally or recreationally.

My investigation revealed at least seven fatal flaws with criminalizing people who use drugs. Together, they convinced me that, as part of a new approach, we need to immediately repeal simple possession of illicit drugs as a criminal offence. These fatal flaws are as follows.

1. Punishing people for having substance use disorders

"The impact of all these drugs being illegal is, of course, causing harm to addicts—and it's all based on our traditional assumption that being an addict is a crime, so it's a bad thing and it should be punished," said Judge Elisabeth Burgess. "But if you look at people who are using [illicit drugs] now, you'd have to be dead yourself not to care about the harm it's caused to the people. We're forcing people underground, obviously, because they can't get [them]."

Criminal offences exist to punish blameworthy conduct. But those with opioid use disorder lack the ability to make an effective choice not to engage in this behaviour. Indeed, as we saw in Chapter 3, that's the very definition of opioid use disorder as understood by medical professionals—an inability to stop using on their own, even if they desperately want to and despite the potential negative consequences.

People with substance use disorders deserve our compassion, not our condemnation. They need our love, respect, and understanding, not the full weight of the state crashing down on them when they're at their lowest low. The pain and suffering in their lives is real and in some cases unimaginable. But our criminal laws ignore all this and also don't deter people from using. As we'll see, they just drive people towards riskier drug use.

Remember the role played by genetics and factors like childhood trauma in opioid use disorder? Trauma such as that experienced by the survivors of residential schools and the Sixties Scoop. Trauma such as that experienced by the Indigenous children who saw their own mother murdered and were left with her body for days. Trauma that, for most, is unfathomable.

Indeed, our laws prohibiting opioid use go back to 1884, a time that pre-dates modern understanding of brain function and addiction. We now know that habitual use of these substances is a medical—not a moral—issue. Our laws need to be updated to reflect that reality.

"It makes no sense to arrest somebody who has a medical problem and often a mental health problem along with it and a whole bunch of other things," said Dr. Bonnie Henry, BC's chief medical officer.

"Many, many families have seen their loved ones be incarcerated for accessing or possessing the drugs they need to not withdraw. That's just wrong. Wrong on all levels," said Leslie McBain.

And the criminal justice system doesn't just punish people for drug possession; in a wide range of offences it also routinely imposes conditions that require people to abstain from using illicit drugs altogether. And for someone with a substance use disorder, an abstinence order is an unrealistic, even impossible demand, one that only sets them up for failure. When they use again or relapse and breach those conditions they're hit with a new offence, typically leading to even greater punishment. It's a cascading effect that leads to a potentially endless cycle of criminalization with no way out—at tremendous cost to taxpayers as well as the person whose life is now firmly entrenched in the criminal justice system. And if they do somehow manage to respect a court abstinence order, their reduced tolerance puts them at significantly greater risk of dying when they do eventually relapse.

A stunning 70% of federal offenders are admitted to prison with serious alcohol and drug abuse problems; 34% of these were injection drug users prior to being incarcerated. Our prisons have become holding facilities for those with mental health issues, substance use disorders, and Indigenous people. Canada's criminal justice system is failing on multiple levels—and a big part of that stems from criminal- izing people who use drugs. As Jordan Westfall, president of the Canadian Association of People Who Use Drugs, told me, "A lot of people get pushed in, not on drug charges, but they get pre-trial con- ditions or bail charges. Stuff like that. . . . That whole aspect of the criminal justice system needs to be reformed because it just leads people into like a cycle of going in and out, in and out. It's just entirely needless."

2. Fuelling stigma

"As long as it's criminal, it's something to do in shame, in private, not to tell anyone," said Jennifer Breakspear. "Hiding is what's going to drive people to do it in secret. Do it where there's no one around to help them. As long as it's illegal, people are afraid to share that piece of themselves and therefore afraid to get any help. No one knows to give them the help."

Sociologists believe that stigma flows from three main sources: family and friends, social agencies, and laws and governmental poli- cies. Indeed, the Supreme Court of Canada has recognized that all criminal offences generate stigma—that is, being labelled by the state and the community with "moral opprobrium," meaning contempt, condemnation, shame, disgrace, and humiliation. Is that really the message the law should be sending to people with substance use disorders in the twenty-first century? That they're worthless and deserving of our vitriol?

"I do believe that stigma drives a lot of this underground," said Clayton Pecknold, assistant deputy minister and director of police services in BC. "I think it also colours the way the broader community sometimes looks at this. I think there's a horrible sector of society that sometimes thinks that people are expendable, that it's their fault they're addicted. They couldn't be more wrong."

"The stigma and discrimination impacts you in so many different ways," said Westfall. "Our government talks about wanting to destigmatize, but you can't really do that—it's still a criminal act at the end of the day. Until they address that, no stigma effort, no poster campaign is going to make a difference."

3. Endangering health and lives

"There's really good literature that shows pretty clearly that the risk of criminal sanctions leads to people using in kind of clandestine ways, and the biggest risk factor for overdose is people using alone," said Dr. Evan Wood. "At the individual level, [a charge for] possession— I think it's counterproductive because it doesn't do anything to stop people from using and it just changes behaviour in terms of riskier use."

This is the deadly consequence of criminalization: driving people to use illicit substances alone, thereby putting them at a substantially greater risk of dying from an overdose. That includes both regular users who have opioid use disorder and people who occasionally or recreationally use illicit drugs. "If you're living in a place where you think someone might call the police on you because you're using drugs, that further stigmatizes that individual," said Dr. Bonnie Henry.

"It puts them underground. It puts them at risk for overdose and death. So that's where it concerns me."

"They don't want to come forward. They're basically hiding," said Westfall. "They're dying inside and alone a lot of times. We talk about ways to get people out? Well, it's illegal. Of course people are going to use by themselves in the relative safety of their own homes."

There are also concerns that homeless people who don't have an indoor residence engage in riskier activity—for example, quickly taking their entire hit rather than progressively dosing up—out of fear of police involvement. "There's lots of literature showing how people will rush and take high risk," said Dr. Wood. "They don't want to have an interaction with law enforcement when using on the streets, or the same thing with not wanting to have negative interaction with the street predators. They use in a rushed way. It just really doesn't achieve its intended effect and obviously has unintended consequences."

There are other concrete ways that our criminal justice system and laws are running afoul of the best medical evidence about how to treat people with opioid use disorder. A classic example is with respect to "drug paraphernalia," which includes sterile syringes. Most courts have something called a "pick list" for lawyers and judges to use in coming up with standardized conditions to impose on accused persons and offenders while they're at large in the community. The BC Provincial Court's most recent pick list includes the following suggestion: "You must not possess drug paraphernalia including but not limited to pipes, rolling papers and syringes." That's problematic for several reasons.

As a Pivot Legal Society representative put it, "Knowing after decades and decades that harm reduction works—and that we can stop the spread of HIV and hepatitis C by provision of clean syringes and by doing needle exchange programs and needle distribution programs—and you're still allowed to tell somebody, 'You're not allowed to hold drug paraphernalia'? And that includes harm reduction equipment that people need, like clean syringes." The prohibition on possessing drug paraphernalia would even punish someone for having a take-home naloxone kit, which contains syringes—something that could save their life or the life of someone overdosing nearby in an emergency. "It's at odds with public health efforts. It means that police officers can literally be like 'Thanks, Health, for spending millions to make sure people have the harm reduction they need. We're just going to confiscate them.'"

Additionally, Canada's federal Good Samaritan Drug Overdose Act (which we looked at in Chapter 9) doesn't protect people from being punished for possessing drug paraphernalia (e.g., syringes) when they're under such a court-ordered prohibition for charges other than simple drug possession (e.g., theft). That clearly needs to change. Many U.S. states include exemptions for drug paraphernalia in their Good Samaritan laws.

Finally, as we saw in Chapter 10, a mountain of evidence supports making supervised consumption sites more widespread. The only reason they require Health Canada approval is the existence of the drug possession offence. In other words, the criminal offence of simple possession of illicit drugs presents an impediment to providing life-saving medical interventions. And as a result there are still far too few of these sites—a fact that has spurred some provinces, like BC and Ontario, to approve their own overdose prevention sites, effectively ignoring federal laws in order to save lives.

4. Isolating people who use drugs from support
Criminalizing those who use drugs cuts them off from receiving support. This can happen in myriad ways, including incarceration. While in jail, those who use illicit drugs (which are still accessible in prisons)

don't have equal access to medical interventions and quality addiction treatment options. They should—especially if one of our goals is that they rehabilitate. Coroners' inquests in both BC and Ontario have flagged this as a major problem, one that's putting people at risk of dying from illicit overdoses while they're imprisoned and upon their eventual release. It's also now the subject of lawsuits arguing that failing to provide inmates with access to harm reduction services (like clean syringes) puts their health at risk and is discriminatory, contrary to the Charter.

Another example of how criminalization cuts people off from support is "red zoning," or the imposition of geographic restrictions, often on those who are released "on conditions." These red zones banish people from a certain area, typically in the vicinity where they allegedly committed an offence or are seen as being a nuisance. However, these same areas can include support services that may keep them alive. But if they enter the red zone they'll face more serious criminal penalties.

"For us, it puts our lives into chaos," said Westfall. "It polices where people can go in certain places, like red zoning so people aren't able to access healthcare or go to Insite or use an overdose prevention site, because it might be on the same block that they're red zoned at. Stuff like this, it just complicates things for us trying to access all kinds of services."

5. Fostering other criminal and risky behaviours

For many people who have opioid use disorder, finding enough money to pay for illicit drugs is a costly and risky proposition. They're charged monopoly prices and they have to deal with drug traffickers, who can be predatory and violent. In Chapter 11, we saw that the patients in the NAOMI project were spending an average of US$1200 per month on street drugs before the study—that's 2.5 times what monthly income assistance provides—and that's not accounting for the money needed for food, shelter, or clothing.

To generate the income to pay drug dealers, some people who are addicted to opioids turn to property crime and prostitution, and even become street-level dealers themselves (reportedly getting one hit as payment for every ten they sell, according to a criminal defence lawyer I interviewed). Property theft typically generates a 10 to 20% return, meaning money paid to dealers generated from stolen goods is just the tip of the iceberg in terms of the cost of prohibition to society. It's one of the likely reasons why thefts from vehicles have skyrocketed in Vancouver in recent years.

Judge Burgess has sentenced homeless people with opioid addictions who've stolen items costing $8000 from luxury stores like Holt Renfrew only to sell them in open-air markets for as low as $10 (the street price for a "half point" or 0.05 grams of heroin). "These people are struggling—and a lot of them are addicts and a lot of them, you know, they cause problems in the community," she told me. "They steal incessantly, and businesses shouldn't have to deal with that, but you can't just take that in isolation and punish them for it."

"The fact that a substance is criminalized and use of that substance is criminalized—it leads to behaviours and identities of people being criminalized," said Chris Buchner. "You see people who are living the most traumatic, violent lives, and people often think, 'That's what happens if you use drugs.' No. That's what happens if you're dependent on a substance that makes you a criminal—and then your whole life and identity and behaviour is criminalized, and you have no access to resources and jobs."

6. Increasing the risk of overdose death upon release from prison
We saw in Chapter 7 that those who've recently been released from

prison are at significantly greater risk of overdosing and dying owing to their reduced tolerance to illicit opioids. The corrections system is actually setting people up for reoffending and a premature death—and this after they've already "paid their debt" to society.

"For opioid dependent inmates released from a correctional facility, they would be provided a prescription for Suboxone to be filled in the community. If an inmate was released from court, they would not return to the correctional facility and may end up being released without a prescription," wrote Michael Egilson, the presiding coroner who investigated Brandon Jansen's death. "When inmates were released, they had a two-week waiting period to obtain social assistance. For most, that meant not being eligible for Pharmacare, requiring the inmate to pay for the Suboxone. This increased the likelihood that opioid dependent inmates would seek out illicit opioids and engage in criminal activity in order to obtain funds."

"They don't do any treatment while in jail," said Mark Gervin, director of legal services at the UBC Indigenous Community Legal Clinic. "They've got a captive audience and they don't treat them. They don't help them in any form or fashion. Ultimately you keep a guy in jail and he hasn't been able to use heroin, or fentanyl, and he gets back out on the street, the higher the chance that he's going to overdose. Because when he went in he was using X, and his body can no longer tolerate X or even half of X. Then they might go out and, boom, they're dead."

7. Raising barriers to rehabilitation

"We need to get people in recovery, and if you criminalize you're basically cutting the opportunity for any of those people to recover," said Dr. Mark Tyndall. "If you make it illegal, if you're 30 years old with no teeth and a criminal record, try reintegrating into society. We've really damaged people by thinking we're doing them a favour by being tough on drugs and being a big deterrent. We've really, really destroyed a lot of people's lives."

One of the key objectives of criminal law is rehabilitation of offenders. Yet criminalizing people with substance use disorders makes their journey towards recovery more difficult in numerous ways.

The experience of imprisonment can itself be devastating for someone who's already endured a lifetime of trauma. "If a person goes to jail, then gets out of jail, everything falls apart in terms of housing, in terms of jobs," Leslie McBain told me. "It's a huge thing."

And the significance of a criminal record cannot be understated. It's a real barrier for those seeking jobs that require a clean record. "We definitely need to change policy on the implementation of criminal records associated with drug substances in the past," said Dr. Paul Hasselback. "Once someone is labelled, that precludes access to some of the supports like meaningful employment. Criminal record checks and all sorts of things potentially can limit what the future is going to look like. A lot of people report back that they've tried very hard to lead a drug-free life, but these obstacles they run into actually drive them back into utilization. It's tragic."

In sum, having outstanding criminal charges, warrants, or a criminal record for simple possession of illicit opioids, or for offences related to generating illicit income to fund street drugs, can have far-reaching consequences. It can severely limit job and career opportunities and the ability to travel internationally, and it can contribute to feelings of worthlessness and shame.

———

The combined effect of these seven massive failings is staggering. Not only has the criminalization of those who use illicit drugs been a colossal failure, it's making the opioid crisis even worse. It's costing lives. If we were starting from scratch and looking at various options for dealing with illicit drugs, the status quo—which has no evidence to support it—would be at the bottom of the list.

All these concerns were sending up red flags in my mind. As a law clerk at the Supreme Court of Canada, as chief legal officer in the Prime Minister's Office, and as a tenured law professor, I've reviewed laws for their compliance with the Canadian Charter of Rights and Freedoms. And during my investigation into the opioid crisis, I've learned that the laws that criminalize people who use drugs are increasing the risk of overdose and death in multiple ways—a clear indication that they may violate the Charter and are thus unconstitutional.

I met with the Pivot Legal Society lawyers, who regularly litigate tough cases at the Supreme Court, to ask their opinion. "I think the prohibition on possession is constitutionally suspect," agreed a Pivot representative. "In the climate we're in right now—and with the feed-back we get from folks about the fact that they're necessarily going to use at home alone because they don't want to be apprehended—it's hugely problematic. I don't see how that could not be a constitutional violation. It's constantly a matter of life and death where someone chooses to use."

The Supreme Court has said that because federal laws allow for supervised consumption sites, the harm is reduced. But that was before the opioid crisis, and without much track record in seeing how difficult it is to get such facilities up and running. These sites don't just face the hurdle of getting Health Canada approval; they often face opposition from local communities and governments, too. "There are so many smaller regional areas that don't have supervised consumption, where even talking about supervised consumption is practically illegal," said Pivot. "What we learned from the overdose prevention sites is it takes a tent and a bucket of naloxone—and that's what you do. The exemption process isn't sufficient to meet that need." And so, in the context of these new facts, a Charter challenge to the criminalization of simple possession of illicit drugs is ripe for the making. Absent political leadership, it may well be the courts that ultimately right the wrong of criminalizing people who use drugs, but that possibility seems far off as people's safety and lives continue to be at risk.

———

"When I talk to everybody else in the field, whether it's police or health, we collectively say, 'What else are we not doing? What can we do differently?' And that's when conversations about decriminalization and legalization are really appropriate. I think it's appropriate for a democracy to look at all options," said Staff Sergeant Conor King.

Having seen the futility of punishing people who are addicted to opioids, the police in Vancouver, Victoria, and Surrey say they're no longer actively prosecuting them for simple possession—although there's evidence at the provincial level that people are still being charged with the offence. Yet medical and public health experts, activists, and drug users say it's not enough, and that decriminalization of possession is needed to reduce stigma, reduce barriers to support and treatment, and treat opioid use disorder like any other medical condition.

"I'd say to really deal with the problem we need to decriminalize drugs," said Dr. Mark Tyndall. "We need to have a hard conversation about what damage we're doing to people and society by continuing to criminalize drug use, which we know doesn't stop people from using drugs. It fills our criminal justice system. It just ruins people's lives.

"We don't want to needlessly punish people, but we don't want to start promoting this. We need to still regulate it and tightly control it."

Dr. Bonnie Henry agrees. "Decriminalization of people who use drugs is absolutely, I think, where we need to go."

It's not just the federal criminal law that punishes and ostracizes people who use drugs. You can see the same policy play out at other levels of government, too. "We need to decriminalize everything," said Westfall. "Not just at the federal level, but it needs to be reflected at provincial and local levels as well. We have these anti–harm reduction ordinances and bylaws. Abbotsford had one a couple of years ago. These things basically blunt the impact of any sort of change that happens federally."

Prohibition is a clever deception. It promises to stop something bad but instead causes more harm in its wake. The law has become a fatal stumbling block to those recovering from their illicit drug use. But if simple possession of illicit drugs were no longer a crime, wouldn't more people use drugs?

"I don't see a problem with that, because that's not going to increase use," said Dr. Neil Boyd, a professor of criminology at Simon Fraser University. "It's just going to finally admit that this whole idea of criminalizing drugs is a bit of a mistake. It's a public health problem. It's not a moral issue."

And it's important to point out that decriminalizing illicit drugs and providing people who have opioid use disorder with a "safe supply" aren't the same as legalizing illicit drugs. Legalization would allow anyone of age to purchase illicit drugs. While there are some advocates who'd like to see that policy model adopted, it represented a very small minority of the people I interviewed. There was, however, significant support for decriminalization combined with a safe supply for those who would otherwise use contaminated street drugs.

What about occasional or recreational drug users? Would decriminalization affect them? To start with, it's the regular users—defined by continued drug use despite the risk of negative consequences, including the threat of a criminal record, fine, and imprisonment—who comprise the vast majority of people who are overdosing and dying. They need to be our primary concern. As for occasional or recreational drug users, if the risk of a fatal overdose isn't going to deter them, the threat of a fine and some jail time is unlikely to have any impact. And since criminalization encourages all drug users to use in secret, where they're at greater risk of dying from an overdose, decriminalization makes sense for that group as well.

———

It's not just Canada that's grappling with the question of how to address illicit drugs and the devastating toll they're taking on our society. The vast majority of countries are firmly entrenched in a drug prohibitionist model. How well is that working? The day I started writing this chapter, the United Nations Office on Drugs and Crime (UNODC) released its *World Drug Report 2018*. The report found that drug seizures have massively increased around the world (including a record 91 tons of heroin seized worldwide in just one year). Of course, to respond to this, the production of illicit drugs has hit record levels, according to the UNODC. As more drugs are seized, more are supplied. That's been a major reason for the rise in synthetic illicit drugs made in labs, like fentanyl. And as we saw in Chapter 4, the Iron Law of Prohibition means that the greater the enforcement, the more potent the drugs we're going to continue to see. Experts at the UNODC concluded that the "range of drugs and drug markets are expanding and diversifying as never before." In other words, the global war on drugs amounts to little more than "security theatre"—incredibly costly countermeasures that look like a lot is being done to combat illicit narcotics, while achieving no practical benefits and actually making things worse.

As Jordan Westfall said, we can keep playing this game—we've been playing it for a century—and things will just keep getting worse. And they are. The definition of insanity, it's often said, is doing the same thing over and over and expecting different results. By that metric, drug prohibition is an insane policy. It was developed for the wrong reasons and it doesn't work. It's time to admit that it's a total failure and causing untold harm. And not only does prohibition not work, it's also expensive. It costs taxpayers $116,000 a year to keep someone in federal prison in Canada, yet the return on investment in treatment is a net benefit, reducing both criminal justice and healthcare costs. So the status quo isn't merely ineffective, it's also costly.

The UNODC reported that around the world, 1 in 20 people between 15 and 64 years of age used drugs at least once in the past year. Some 450,000 of them died as a result of drug use in 2015. Fatal drug overdoses are so numerous that, for the first time in half a century, life expectancy in the United States went down for two consecutive years. There's even a drug epidemic underway in Africa with another synthetic opioid, called tramadol. Tomorrow it will be a different substance we won't have heard of until it's too late. Our children and grandchildren are going to grow up and ask us what we were thinking. I have no doubt that history will judge drug prohibition harshly.

Billions upon billions of dollars continue to be spent worldwide on criminal enforcement against illicit drugs, with massive violence in the streets as rival traffickers fight each other for turf and battle against increasingly militarized police forces. Prohibition has fuelled civil wars, corruption, and regional instability. The war on drugs hasn't in the least stopped these substances from reaching the streets, but it has filled prisons across the globe. In the United States it has produced such mass incarceration that half of all federal inmates are imprisoned on drug-related charges. Yet illicit drugs are just as available and more potent than ever. At the same time, fewer than one in six people with drug use disorders are receiving treatment around the world—and that's a generous estimate.

As one global campaign argues, "Support, don't punish"—which is exactly the approach some countries are beginning to take: treating substance use as a health and social issue rather than as a criminal and moral one. It's a relatively new model that's already demonstrated a lot of potential, and that should give Canada the confidence to move ahead in a similar way.

Many of the people I interviewed held up Portugal as an example of a country that has adopted a promising new drug policy. In the late 1990s, in response to an increase in intravenous heroin use and rising rates of infectious diseases, Portugal launched a review of its entire approach to dealing with illicit drugs. Prohibition had failed. It was time for a humane approach to people who use drugs. The aim would be to prevent drug use and abuse by decriminalizing personal drug use and possession, pursuing prevention initiatives, expanding and improving treatment options, and offering treatment instead of imprisonment for drug users.

On July 1, 2001, the Portuguese government took the definitive step of decriminalizing the personal acquisition, possession, and use of small quantities of illicit drugs (including cocaine and heroin), instead making it an administrative offence. Those found in possession of such small quantities are referred within 72 hours to a "Commission for the Dissuasion of Drug Addiction" that includes lawyers, social workers, and medical professionals. If those found in possession aren't dependent on drugs, the commission can provisionally suspend proceedings and order them to take a psychological or educational program; it can impose such sanctions as warnings, community service, suspension of professional licences, and banishment from certain places; or it can require them to pay a fine. If those found in possession *are* dependent on drugs, the commission can recommend a treatment program instead of a sanction. Imprisonment isn't an option. And although Portugal has decriminalized drugs, it did not legalize them to enable public access to illicit drugs. Illicit drug manufacturing and drug trafficking remain crimes.

Has this novel approach worked?

Like every controversial policy change, it has its supporters and its detractors. When I began to read the research on the Portugal model, I quickly discovered two very different narratives. One of the first high-profile reports declared it a "resounding success," but soon afterwards a competing series of blog postings and website articles claimed it to be a "disastrous failure." The former was written by an American constitutional lawyer and published by the CATO Institute, a U.S.-based libertarian think tank founded by Charles G. Koch and funded by the Koch brothers. The latter were written by a drug abstinence–based treatment provider and published by the Association for a Drug Free Portugal. Neither of these accounts appeared in peer-reviewed journals, but they have driven intense international attention and debate about the Portugal model.

I knew I needed to find unbiased, scientifically validated findings. It turns out that there *is* compelling evidence in peer-reviewed journals of the Portugal model's success, on balance. It's not without its blemishes, though. Still, knowing that gives us a more realistic perspective—after all, even the best life-saving medications can have side effects. In order to make an informed decision, we just need to know what they are.

Dr. Caitlin Hughes, a criminologist and research fellow at the National Drug and Alcohol Research Centre at the University of New South Wales (Australia), and Dr. Alex Stevens, a criminal justice professor at the University of Kent (U.K.), did the tough but necessary work of sifting through the competing claims about the Portugal model. Hughes and Stevens found that both sides were guilty of some selective use of data and made claims that weren't supported by the available evidence. As well, given that many factors can affect outcomes, we can't assume that they're entirely attributable to changes in law and policy. But on the whole, Hughes and Stevens's research rejects the fearful speculation that decriminalization will make things worse. Instead, they found that Portugal "may offer a model for other nations that wish to provide less punitive, more integrated and effective responses to drug use."

Most notably, drug-induced deaths declined significantly after decriminalization. The best available data from the National Statistics Institute in Portugal reveals a massive drop: from almost 80 deaths in 2001 to just 20 in 2008, representing an almost 75% reduction in the seven years after decriminalization. And the decline in opioid-related overdose deaths has been a major part of this good news story. Why did it happen?

"The fall in deaths related to opiates has been linked to the big increase in the numbers of heroin users who have entered substitution treatment [such as methadone or buprenorphine], as substitution treatment has repeatedly been found to be effective in reducing the mortality of opiate users. It may also be another indicator of falling levels of heroin use," wrote Hughes and Stevens.

Instead of threatening people with imprisonment, authorities are now connecting them with treatments to help them manage the horrific symptoms of withdrawal. That makes a lot of sense, given what I'd learned about substance use disorders. Drug use is being treated not as a crime but as a health issue.

But what about the broader society? Has decriminalization increased or decreased drug use in Portugal? Sifting through the statistical debates, Hughes and Stevens found that while there appears to have been some short-term increases in drug use by people who were likely experimenting ("lifetime use" rates increased), rates of discontinuance have increased too, meaning that fewer people who've tried drugs are continuing to use them. Between 2001 (when decriminalization began) and 2007, recent and current drug use increased in older age groups but declined in the critical 15- to 24-year-old population (those who are considered harbingers of drug use rates). Overall, these mixed results are seen as a net benefit. And when we look closer at which drugs are involved, the picture becomes more compelling.

There has been a significant reduction in the percentage of people referred to the Commissions for the Dissuasion of Drug Addiction for heroin in the years after decriminalization. In 2001, when these commissions first started receiving referrals as part of the decriminalization framework, 47% of people were referred for cannabis, 33% for heroin, and 5% for cocaine. By 2005, 65% of people were referred for cannabis, 15% for heroin (a more than 50% cut), and 6% for cocaine. It's another indicator that decriminalization hasn't led to an increase in "hard drug" use that some speculated would occur.

There are a few aspects of the Portugal model, however, that suggest we can't simply copy and paste it into Canada and expect the opioid crisis to be solved overnight. First, Portugal did not adopt its approach in the midst of an emergency like our own, one that's been driven by a contaminated illicit drug supply. More will be needed here, particularly in the provision of a "safe" supply of drugs to those who are addicted and would otherwise be at risk of an illicit drug overdose.

Second, we have to be careful not to simply import policy models from other jurisdictions with major economic, social, and cultural differences from our own and expect them to work exactly the same here. For instance, the significant challenges faced by Indigenous Canadians during the opioid crisis require particular attention and a specialized response.

Third, the Portugal model still involves a degree of coercion—if a person who's addicted to illicit drugs isn't willing to enter treatment they can face sanctions, although it's unclear to what extent this is happening in practice. I noted in Chapter 12 that forced treatment doesn't generally work, nor is it consistent with the nature of ongoing illicit drug use as a medical condition. And in some circumstances, Portugal also fines people who use drugs. As I recounted at the start of this chapter, I saw firsthand with my own client, Jim, that fining a street-level drug user is ridiculous: it makes no sense to compel someone to pay a fine that they can't afford and that doesn't prove to be any kind of deterrent.

But although we shouldn't put all our faith in the Portugal model as a panacea for Canada's opioid crisis, the general approach it advocates is promising. Many of the people I interviewed, including some police officers, strongly support its general approach, which combines decriminalizing simple possession of illicit drugs with expanding access to treatment. Those are key building blocks of a compassionate, evidence-based drug policy.

———

Now, at the end of my investigation into the opioid crisis, I'm convinced that we must decriminalize simple possession of illicit drugs and radically change how our criminal justice system and our laws deal with people with opioid use disorder.

It's time to stop punishing those with substance use disorders and instead treat them with compassion. It's time to stop fuelling the stigma that's endangering people's lives and instead help them deal with their pain and trauma. It's time to stop deploying criminal law in ways that run counter to the best medical evidence about opioid use disorder and how to treat it. It's time to stop the endless cycle of criminalization that helps no one and that comes at a massive cost to those who use illicit drugs and to our society as a whole. It's time to stop locking up vast numbers of people with substance use and mental health issues and instead help them get the treatment and support they need. It's time to end the failed experiment of prohibition and the war on drugs.

But getting to this point was a real journey for me. It required an open mind and an open heart. And I hope that sharing my own transformation will help others see the opioid crisis through different eyes.

I'm not alone in experiencing such a shift in outlook. Linda Lupini, executive vice president of the BC Provincial Health Services Authority and BC Emergency Health Services, told me of another example: "We had the head of the paramedic service in Ottawa come and visit us, and he said, 'How are you dealing with this? It's starting to show up in Ontario.' We went and took him on a tour. When we started talking about decriminalization and safe injection sites and overdose prevention sites, he said, 'You guys are really out there. People coming in, injecting. What are you guys talking about?' Anyway, he spent a week here. At the end of the week he came for a debrief and he said, 'I'm a hundred percent supportive of everything you guys do. My mind has been completely turned.'"

But so far, the powers that be haven't been willing to take the controversial step of declaring the war on drugs to be a failure and decriminalizing people who use drugs in order to help save their lives. The federal Liberals and the Conservatives have both balked at the suggestion. As a senior BC provincial official (who requested anonymity) told me, "I've sat in two meetings with the prime minister, and I mean the highest level, with [the now former] Minister of Justice and Attorney General Jody Wilson-Raybould and eight other people—small meetings in Vancouver, two of them. . . . We begged for money and we begged for decriminalization, and we got $10 million sent to the [BC] government after the first meeting. And we were told, directly from the prime minister, it's not happening—decriminalization."

"He said that right to you?" I asked.

"Right to our face. 'It's not happening,' he said. 'You have no idea what I've been through across this country trying to deal with the marijuana and cannabis issue. I can tell you straight out, it's not happening.' Then he came back and said, 'You know, I gave you the $10 million.' And we're like, 'Okay—that's going to help us save more people over the next year, but that's not going to fix this permanently. We need to talk again about decriminalization.'"

This description of a closed-door March 2017 meeting with Prime Minister Justin Trudeau was independently confirmed by Leslie McBain with Moms Stop the Harm, who was also in attendance. "At the end of the meeting we were all asking for decriminalization," she said. "Ending the war on drugs. There were police officers in there, there were front-line emergency response teams, there were doctors, there were social workers, there were people with lived experience, myself. We all had the same message.

"'Well, I hear you and I understand, and I'm sympathetic,'" McBain quoted Trudeau as saying. "'But do you know how much trouble I'm having legalizing pot?'

"We all sat there in stunned silence," she continued. "That was his stance then and that seems to be his stance today. He's almost ignoring it, it seems. It was a nothing response."

These accounts reflect a prime minister who'd faced political challenges with legalizing cannabis and so wouldn't consider decriminalizing hard drugs. In other words, the position he took was entirely political—based neither on evidence during a public health emergency nor on the advice of the experts he met with. I wrote to Trudeau asking for his own account of the meeting, and never received a reply.

Lives being lost in this ongoing crisis are the equivalent of a fully-loaded large passenger aircraft crashing and killing everyone aboard every 5 to 6 weeks in Canada. Yet it didn't even merit a mention during the 2019 federal election leaders' debate or make it onto the CBC's list of election issues.

"If that doesn't break the shell and get into the psyche of the government, what will?" asked McBain. "We're getting small funding here, small funding there. And it's good, we need it, but the big things that need to be done are not being done. We haven't declared a national state of health emergency, and we haven't seen anyone in the upper echelons of government talk about the fact that we need to take these courageous moves to stop the deaths."

$-14-$

HOW CAN WE
SOLVE THIS CRISIS?

Troy Balderson apologized for running late. A water leak had sprung that morning at one of the shelters run by Lookout Housing and Health Society in Vancouver's Downtown Eastside, which also runs the Powell Street Getaway supervised consumption site. Balderson is the charitable organization's downtown projects manager. He had a lot on his plate, but the leak wasn't a problem that fazed him. Not long before it was six people overdosing in a single night in one of their buildings. That put the other trials of his job in perspective.

"We understand that everybody comes from a past, and we're not here to put barriers between them and our services," said Balderson. We were sitting in his small office, filled with boxes of supplies, near the shelter's busy entrance. The Powell Street Getaway also provides meals, medication administration, emergency clothing, social activities, and employment and internship programs as well as substance use and mental health programs. "We meet them where they're at."

"What do you think needs to be done to really address this crisis?" I asked.

"If we get enough people to understand that it's not just a bunch of druggies shooting drugs," he explained. "That it's people suffering from many, many stages of trauma, from many, many walks of life.

"They're invisible. If we take the time to speak with those folks, that's all it takes. It's a simple hello. A simple 'I'm going to take five minutes out of my day. I'm going to spend it with you and you're going to be heard.' That in itself is probably a bigger gift than anybody knows. Just taking that time."

Balderson's words stayed with me as I stepped back from months of speaking with people on the front lines of the opioid crisis. It was now crystal clear to me: our response to this epidemic must begin with care and compassion for those who, for many reasons, have come to self-medicate the physical, psychological, and emotional pain and trauma in their lives using illicit opioids. That means no longer essentially criminalizing opioid use disorder but instead ensuring that people have safe places to use substances of known contents and potency. It means developing connections with them as a prelude to offering rapid access to evidence-based treatment options if and when they want to stop using.

As we've seen, Canada's century-long experiment with drug prohibition and tough-on-crime drug policies has been a miserable failure. The opioid crisis has exposed the war on drugs as a fundamentally flawed response to the risks associated with illegal drugs. And it's not just Canada that's following this wrongheaded and punitive approach to dealing with drug users.

I couldn't believe how far I'd come over the last 100 days: the things I'd seen and heard about, the people I'd met along the way. My mind had changed and my heart had expanded. A few years ago you couldn't have paid me to wear a T-shirt that declared "End the War on Drugs"; now I wanted to order a caseload and distribute them myself. My investigation into the opioid crisis that started in my hometown of Vancouver had opened my eyes to a totally different reality. In retrospect, my previous views about illegal drugs were based on ignorance and ideology—a dangerous combination. Critically, they weren't evidence-based—informed by medical or criminology research, let alone the actual experiences of people who use drugs.

And a remarkable thing happened as I began sharing my findings with people: they started opening up, too. When I talked about decriminalization to a friend of mine, an emergency room physician, it turned out that he was totally supportive of it. An old friend from university revealed that his girlfriend was addicted to heroin and that he was grateful for the research I was doing. My investigation has given me a better understanding of some of the challenges that people who use drugs are facing, although I'll never fully appreciate what their day-to-day challenges are like.

I've come to see that there's a clear moral wrong in this whole issue: the injustice of unmercifully judging and punishing people who are using drugs in an attempt to get relief from the pain in their lives. As I've studied, thought about, and prayed about this issue all along the way, that's a truth I've come to understand not only at an intellectual but also at a spiritual level. It's been a real transformation. I was dead wrong about drug policy. Our response to substance use must be one of care, compassion, and understanding for those who are using. We're in no place to judge and condemn them. Rather, we're called to love them. And establishing that loving connection can help bring hope for a better future—something crucial for addiction recovery that can't be obtained through a prescription.

I went back to the list of questions I'd written up at the beginning of my investigation. Reading them again, it was clear that many were based on myths and stereotypes that I'd now thoroughly debunked based on my research.

The promise of prohibition was a lie—a quixotic, aspirational policy that's not only unrealistic but dangerous. I'd have a much harder time purchasing unpasteurized milk in Vancouver than I would purchasing illicit drugs. Why? Because milk sales are regulated and subject to rigorous health and safety standards, whereas illicit drugs have zero oversight. Instead of stopping drugs, as it promised, prohibition has left the drug market as a "free-for-all" to be run completely by organized crime—they make their illicit products without any standards and are almost never held accountable when people die as a result.

Show me the peer-reviewed research that says prohibition works. You couldn't design a worse approach to substance use disorder if you tried. What an insane system we've come to accept "for the good of society." Prohibition isn't good for society; it's been a disaster. The first step in coming up with a new approach is admitting it, and ending our collective denial and apathy.

The threat of criminal sanctions doesn't deter those with opioid use disorder from seeking out and using illicit drugs, but it compels them to use alone where they're at greater risk of dying in the event of an overdose. And, for people who might be thinking of experimenting with street drugs, the distant prospect of criminal penalties for possession are nowhere near as discouraging as the ever-present risk of suffering a fatal overdose. The experience of Portugal in decriminalizing drugs is very promising, notably in reducing illicit drug overdose deaths and expanding treatment options. We need to fundamentally shift the starting point of our drug policy so that it's understood to be not a criminal matter but rather a public health, medical, and social issue.

———

Prevention should also be part of the response to illicit drug use, but it needs to be done right. Lisa Lapointe, chief coroner with the

BC Coroners Service, cites research finding that "interactive, skills-based approaches showed positive results, with targeted approaches being especially effective."

What *hasn't* been found helpful is fear-mongering. "Evidence suggests that the reasons for drug use are complex and multifaceted, and programs focused on scaring people from using drugs are not effective in saving lives," Lapointe writes. "Additionally, they tend to increase the stigma surrounding drug use and actually discourage people from seeking help—an obsolete approach that has led to the loss of countless lives."

This applies to young people as well. Lapointe cites the massive "Just Say No" and D.A.R.E. campaigns undertaken by the U.S. government to discourage youth from using illicit drugs—initiatives with a US$1 billion total price tag that were later found to have had "no positive effects on youth behaviour and may have, in fact, prompted some to actually experiment with using substances."

We live in a lovely family neighbourhood in East Vancouver, a few blocks from a busy street. There are lots of great restaurants and small grocery stores, but you'll also occasionally see used syringes in the tall grass beside the sidewalk near the thoroughfare. So we had to educate our children about staying out of the grass there and about what syringes were—to not touch them since it's not safe, and to let an adult know if they come across any. It was also an opportunity to talk about drug use. One thing I'd already learned about kids is that telling them not to do something is the fastest way to make them do that thing. Same as with us adults, probably.

"Some people use drugs because they're sad and want to feel better, then they can't stop," I said to my young kids. "But the drugs can hurt them and make things even worse." Then I let them ask questions and answered them as best as I could.

"Kids need to get age-appropriate information on drugs and addiction. Especially the middle school and high schoolers—they must have current, continually updated information on drug safety," said Leslie McBain. "If we want to look a little more long-term than next month or next year, kids have to start to understand themselves, their own anxieties, their own fears. Things that would make them want to try a drug to feel better. And also the dangers of just experimenting."

Research has found that having higher self-esteem, supportive relationships with adults, and positive role models helps youth engage in less substance use. And as McBain says, giving them the facts about substance use in a sensitive, nonjudgmental manner is key. This includes the fact that fentanyl can be fatal if consumed, and how difficult it is to know whether it's present in illegal drugs.

Here are some other tips from the experts about how to talk to youth about substance use:

- Educate yourself so you can answer questions. If you don't know the answers, offer to look for them together.
- Become informed. Learn about the substances commonly used by young people. Find out how the substances work, what their street names are, and the signs of being under the influence.
- Be a good listener. Give your kids room to participate and ask questions. Respect their opinion.
- Stick to the facts. Avoid preaching, scare tactics and exaggeration. Research shows these tactics do not work, and may actually lead to a loss of trust.
- Look for natural opportunities to discuss substance use and decision-making, including stories in the news and social media.

- Be open and respectful. Ask questions about what they're hearing, seeing, or have learned. Then, listen. Talk about why people use substances and the potential consequences.
- Focus on your heartfelt concerns for their safety and a deep regard for their wellness (in contrast to right/wrong, good/bad, obey/punish). Emphasize your deep caring and commitment to understand in contrast to setting them straight.

———

In the face of the scale and complexity of the opioid crisis, it's easy to think that we have little power to effect change. But when we see suffering and injustice, one of the most important things we can do is respond to it directly. Here are 10 concrete actions you can take today to help address the opioid crisis.

1. Tell someone.
Among the biggest impediments to a more compassionate, evidence-based drug policy is a lack of knowledge and the prevalence of stereotypes. Truth will always be a powerful force for those who are able to hear it and are willing to speak it. Share this book and what you've learned with a family member, friend, or colleague. Many of them probably have the same questions I did when I started on this journey. Some of them have probably been affected by the opioid crisis or know someone who has been.

2. Show your support for a compassionate, evidence-based drug policy.
One way to demonstrate this support is by sharing my Vancouver Declaration on Responding to the Opioid Crisis, which summarizes

the main policy and legal recommendations in this book. It appears in the Appendix that follows, and can be found at www.overdosebook.ca.

Some of these recommendations can have an immediate impact, whether in directly saving lives or in reducing the risks faced by people who use drugs. Others will take time to bear fruit. But the evidence is clear: they will benefit not only those who use drugs but also their family members, friends, and society as a whole. It's taken over a century to get into this mess, and it will likely take a generation or more to make substantial progress in getting out of it. We have to start now.

3. Learn how to save a life.

Take the free online training course on how to provide emergency first aid in the event of a drug overdose at www.naloxonetraining .com. It takes only 10 to 15 minutes to learn how to save a life. As we've seen throughout this book, you never know when you may encounter someone who's experiencing a drug overdose. Ask that this training be included in the health and safety training where you work, go to school, or volunteer. You never know when you might need it.

4. Get a take-home naloxone kit.

Once you've taken the online training course, get one of these kits— which, depending on where you live, may be available at your local pharmacy. Keep it secure, close by in your purse, backpack, or computer bag. You might feel nervous about getting one. Think about why that is. It's the stigma of someone thinking you're a drug user. Remember: you're asking for something that could save the life of someone you know and love. Be a hero, just like Little Doug Nickerson.

5. Love and support friends and family members who use drugs.

Show friends and family members who use drugs your love and help them get into treatment when they're willing and able. Connect with support groups in your community or a national group like Leslie McBain's Moms Stop the Harm (www.momsstoptheharm.com) so that they can support you. It's not going to be easy, but getting support from others who've walked this difficult path can make a big difference. Make sure friends or family members who use drugs know about tips for "safer use," as suggested by medical experts. These include the following:

- It is important that help (9-1-1) is called immediately in the event of an overdose;
- Do not use alone (use drugs in an overdose prevention site or supervised consumption site where possible; have someone nearby who can call for help);
- Get trained in overdose response and have naloxone available;
- Start low (test a small amount of the drug) and go slow;
- Know your tolerance: if recently using less drugs or feeling unwell, use less of the drug; and
- Don't mix drugs, or drugs with alcohol.

6. Raise awareness.

Host an awareness-raising event with your friends, work associates, church, synagogue, mosque, temple, or service club to tell them about the opioid crisis and commit together to doing something to address the problem. Reach out to people who have experience with substance use, and include them. We need to go from individual awareness and action to community-based awareness and action.

7. Help get our political leaders on board.

As we saw in the last chapter, one of the main reasons for inaction on the opioid crisis is a lack of political will. Politicians work for you and me. You're their boss, and they typically want to keep their jobs. Make sure they know you care about this issue and won't accept drug policies based on ignorance, fear, ideology, and stereotypes. Write, call, email, and social media message the political leaders in your community at the municipal, provincial, and federal levels to ask them to publicly support the recommendations in the Vancouver Declaration on Responding to the Opioid Crisis. It's also sometimes helpful to focus on one concrete change you especially want to see happen.

8. Speak up.

Raise this issue in letters to the editor, on social media, at political debates, in the classroom or workplace, and at town hall meetings. There's a real risk that people will simply forget about it, moving on to the next perceived crisis of the moment or cute cat meme.

9. Donate your time or money.

Donate your time or money to local groups in your community that are working to help people with substance use disorders, or groups working to help address related issues such as homelessness, mental health issues, or childhood trauma. Non-profit organizations need your help, since many of these services have been chronically under-funded for decades. That's one of the reasons why the opioid crisis has hit so hard. Wherever we have the means to help out, no matter how little, we should.

10. Make a career out of it.

Consider making a career out of helping the millions of people in North America who are struggling with substance use disorders.

There are a growing number of post-secondary education and job opportunities in the field. Or, just as I'm trying to do here, think of how you can do something to help in your existing job, volunteer positions, or circles of influence. There are people you can reach that no one else can. Achieving lasting change requires people with all kinds of unique talents and gifts. Don't underestimate your ability to be part of the solution. Be creative.

———

How does the opioid crisis end? Unless we do something radically different to stem the tide, the realistic worst-case scenario is that overdose death rates decline because there are fewer and fewer people who use drugs left alive, month after month, year after year. In that catastrophic scenario, illicit opioid use will eventually abate by raw attrition. Crisis averted. And we'll all go back to our regularly scheduled programming—except for the tens of thousands of friends, family, and loved ones left behind. That's what I fear will happen if apathy and numb acceptance of massive overdose death rates become the new normal—and if prejudice, ignorance, and crass political considerations prevail over research, evidence, and a heart of compassion for people affected by this unnatural disaster.

Dr. Ronald Joe, medical director for substance use services at Vancouver Coastal Health, remarked to me that, with so many deaths among opioid users, one had to wonder whether it might stop only after everyone had died. "That's not a very good endgame," he said. "No one wishes that. We definitely do not wish that, but I could say that the thought is in our minds." Of course, the threat of a poisoned drug supply remains a deadly hazard for new, occasional, or casual users, too.

In the midst of the despair, destruction, and death that has characterized the opioid crisis, is there any hope? This was the final unanswered question I had—and the one that almost everyone who read the manuscript had. Beyond the public health interventions, latest pharmaceutical treatments, social programs, and legal reforms, could this crisis abate? And even if we're able to keep more people alive, is there any hope that people can be ultimately freed from addiction's chains?

"Addiction doesn't occur in needles and spoons and lighters and bottles and whatnot. Addiction occurs in the brain," said Marshall Smith, senior advisor for recovery initiatives at the British Columbia Centre on Substance Use. "No matter what the substance is that people are using out there, this is a people problem. This is a crisis of community. It's a crisis of connection and it's a crisis that's occurring in people, in families, in workplaces. We like to simplify that and say that it's an opiate problem and point the finger at the drug as if it's the bad thing, and that's just not the case."

Having hope for a better future is vital in overcoming despair. Indeed, without hope, people perish. Alone and without hope, people are continuing to die in large numbers during this epidemic. But there's no prescription for hope. It doesn't come in a pill. You can't manufacture it.

"You know what gets you through? Number one is the community. It's just having support. The second is faith," said Bill Mollard, president of Union Gospel Mission. "When you talk to most of the people out on the streets, they all have faith. And how else could you live on the street? So there is a faith component out there. People are saying 'I need something to believe in that's on my side and willing to help me.' And then they'll begin to look at it."

Finding hope through faith resonated with me. But I wanted to know whether there was any research that would support what Mollard was saying about his personal experience working in Vancouver's Downtown Eastside.

Dr. Alexandre Laudet, director of the Center for the Study of Addictions and Recovery in New York, has investigated the role of faith in the struggle against addiction. "Human beings have long looked to faith for strength and support, particularly in difficult times," she writes. "Scientific research and clinical practice were slow to acknowledge and to investigate the role of this dimension of the human experience, in large part because it is not easily defined or captured using traditional quantitative measures."

Dr. Laudet notes that in recent decades there have been over 200 studies demonstrating the positive role played by faith in mental adjustment and better health. It's been found to support greater emotional well-being and improved coping by giving people hope and strength to deal with stressful events. And there's an increasing interest in the role that faith can play in addressing addiction.

"A growing body of empirical research supports the notion that religiousness and spirituality may enhance the likelihood of attaining and maintaining recovery from addictions, and recovering persons often report that religion and/or spirituality are critical factors in the recovery process," Dr. Laudet writes. "The hope for a better life that sets many substance users on the path to recovery can be a reality."

Recovery can be a life-changing transformation for people emerging from years or even decades of addiction. Since addiction has provided temporary relief from the pain and suffering in their life, being in recovery means finding new and healthy ways to deal with those feelings. Addiction has robbed them of genuine connections to the people around them, and may have disrupted their spiritual connection as well. Indeed, as Dr. Laudet puts it, some "substance users often come into recovery feeling abandoned by God or alienated from God or from the religious community." And yet a new life is possible.

"Being in recovery has changed the way I see God. I came into recovery with a God, but it was a punishing, vengeful and unforgiving God. I had done so many things . . . I knew were ungodly, that I thought for sure I was going to Hell," said Craig, a 44-year old in recovery. "When I came into recovery I found a new God. I found a God that was loving, forgiving, understanding and responsive to the need that I have. In retrospect, I can see that God has been with me all the time."

A study of 14 countries (including Canada) by the World Health Organization found that people with drug addiction had the highest level of social disapproval or stigma of any class of individual—worse even than those with leprosy. That gave me real pause as I remembered back to why I started looking into the opioid crisis in the first place—a prayer to God for a heart of compassion for people affected by it. The same Jesus who I follow laid his hands on people with leprosy when no one else would even come near them. Are more professing Christians willing to similarly love and care for people who use drugs, rather than judge and condemn them? A diverse coalition, including people who use drugs, families and friends affected by the opioid crisis, health and medical practitioners, Indigenous communities, human rights advocates, liberals, progressives, fiscal conservatives, libertarians, and people of faith, need to be part of a major societal shift in how we think about and deal with substance use.

Each of us is on our own unique journey in life, but we're not alone. It's being increasingly acknowledged that the opposite of addiction is connection. When important relationships in our life are disrupted or never fully developed, it causes pain and suffering and makes it more difficult to cope with all the stress, challenges, and trauma of this world. Substances and unhealthy behaviours may appear to soothe that pain temporarily, but are ultimately self-destructive. That path leads to isolation, shame, and despair. Our society often makes it worse by heaping judgment and blame on top of that brokenness. The other path is totally different. It is one of connection, love, and hope. The first path leads to death, the other to life.

Many of the courageous people who are leading the effort to address the opioid crisis and whom I got to know through this book are themselves in recovery from substance use disorders. Today they're leading recovery centres, running safe consumption sites, and acting as powerful advocates for change. They're living full, satisfying lives. And each of them in their own way has found hope and is living free from the chains of addiction. What's most remarkable is that they're now supporting others in their journey of recovery. They're sharing the love that was poured into their lives in order to help others who can hardly dare to imagine one day being free.

APPENDIX

I wrote the Declaration that follows as a way to summarize the book's main legal and policy recommendations in a clear and concise format that could be helpful for those who want to advocate for a more compassionate, evidence-based drug policy. I named it the Vancouver Declaration on Responding to the Opioid Crisis not only because it's the city that's been hardest hit in Canada by the opioid crisis, but also because it's the city that's been at the forefront of courageous and innovative responses to it. Fittingly, I finished drafting this Declaration the morning of July 1, 2018—Canada Day.

It doesn't include everything that could or should be done to address the crisis, but instead focuses on the most significant proposals that would have the greatest immediate to mid-term impact. If you want to show your support for these life-saving ideas, you can visit www.overdosebook.ca, share it on social media, and call on your elected officials and community leaders to publicly declare their support for it too.

Vancouver Declaration on
Responding to the Opioid Crisis

Whereas all people have the right to life, liberty, and security of the person, yet thousands of Canadians have lost their lives to illicit drug overdose;

Whereas the opioid crisis is a public health emergency;

Whereas opioid use disorder is a chronic, relapsing condition affecting thousands of Canadians;

Whereas the majority of people who are dying from illicit drug overdose are using alone and stigma is contributing to them doing so;

Whereas Indigenous people and people released from custody have been disproportionately affected by fatal overdoses;

Whereas drug use is a health and social issue, not a criminal issue;

Whereas over a century of drug prohibition has failed to meet its objectives and it has instead created a lucrative underground market for illicit drugs with significant harm to individuals, families, communities, and nations;

Whereas criminalizing people who use drugs has exacerbated the opioid crisis by punishing people for having substance use disorders, fuelling stigma, endangering their health and lives, isolating them from support, fostering other criminal and risky behaviours, increasing the risk of overdose death upon release from prison and for years later, and raising barriers to rehabilitation;

Whereas drug laws and policies should be based on evidence and compassion for people who are using drugs—not ignorance, fear, ideology, and stereotypes;

Therefore, we call on all levels of government, health authorities and medical practitioners, criminal justice and corrections professionals, and civil society to do everything within their power to:

1. Make **naloxone** freely and widely available to individuals, and at public and private locations, and provide emergency first aid training in how to respond to an overdose;

2. Immediately expand, and remove all legal barriers to, **supervised consumption sites**, overdose prevention sites, witnessed-use rooms, and "no-questions asked" **drug testing** services in all affected communities;

3. Dramatically expand rapid access to **evidence-based treatment** as recommended in the new national guidelines for treating opioid use disorder, including Suboxone as a first-line treatment option;

4. Provide **legal, low-barrier, regulated access to opioids of known contents and potency ("safe supply")**, under medical direction and supervision (e.g., diacetylmorphine, hydromorphone, and extended release medications) to people with opioid use disorder who would otherwise use contaminated street drugs and be at greater risk of a fatal overdose;

5. Invest in **research to develop new treatment options** for opioid use disorder and a **holistic response** to responding to substance use disorders;

6. Increase **support to Indigenous communities, front-line and peer-based organizations, and families** of people with opioid use disorder so that they can enhance their response to the opioid crisis;

7. **Stop criminalizing people who use drugs**, including:
    a. **Expand Good Samaritan overdose laws** to include immunity from prosecution for any non-violent offence and related breaches of conditions and warrants, as well as increase awareness of this legal protection;

b. **Decriminalize simple possession** of illicit drugs;

c. **Cease imposing drug paraphernalia prohibitions**, which prevent the possession of naloxone kits and harm reduction supplies like clean syringes;

d. Stop criminal law conditions that prohibit people from using illicit substances (**"abstinence orders"**);

e. End the imposition of geographic restrictions (**"red zoning"**) of people who use drugs;

f. Make substance use disorder a **mitigating factor at sentencing**;

g. **Expunge criminal records** for possession of illicit substances;

h. **Provide people in prison with equal access** to overdose prevention services, harm reduction supplies, and evidence-based treatment options; and

i. **Prior to their release from custody**, provide people with access to a medical practitioner who is trained in substance use disorders and who can provide them with the necessary information and medications to reduce their risk of suffering a fatal overdose.

METHODOLOGY

For the geeks (I admit to being one) and the skeptics (I used to be one), here's a brief word about how I conducted my investigation. My research involved a mixed-methods approach. Given the emergent nature of the opioid crisis, in addition to conducting a thorough literature review on the subject, my primary sources of information for this study derived from empirical research, using qualitative methods.

Forty-two individuals with expertise related to the opioid crisis were interviewed using a semi-structured method for between 45 and 90 minutes each. These individuals are listed in the Interviewees section. Most interviews were conducted in person in Vancouver, Surrey, and Victoria between February and April 2018, with a few additional interviews in May and June 2018. Where in-person interviews weren't possible they were conducted by telephone. All interviews were digitally recorded, with the permission of the participant, and transcribed by a professional transcription service. The interview transcripts were analyzed using thematic analysis, supported by Nvivo 11 software.

All interviews were conducted with the written informed consent of participants and with harmonized ethics approval from the UBC Behavioural Research Ethics Board, Vancouver Coastal Health Research Institute, Providence Health Care, Fraser Health, and Island Health. Operational approval was also secured from these health authorities. The interviews were for attribution, unless the participant wished to be anonymous.

Additional primary sources were consulted, including to check facts from the interviews, such as public court records, archival sources, judicial decisions, coroner's reports, and records released under the BC Freedom of Information and Protection of Privacy Act. Secondary sources included legal, criminological, sociological, medical, addiction, and public health peer-reviewed literature as well as governmental and non-governmental reports. Specific written sources that I relied upon in the book appear in the Notes section.

INTERVIEWEES

*In alphabetical order, titles/positions listed
at time of being interviewed*

Daniel Atkinson Deputy Fire Chief for Operations, Victoria Fire Department

Shawna Baher Inspector, Surrey RCMP Detachment

Troy Balderson Downtown Projects Manager, Lookout Society

Dr. Aamir Bharmal Medical Health Officer & Medical Director of Communicable Diseases and Harm Reduction, Fraser Health

Oren Bick Senior Counsel, Public Prosecution Service of Canada

Sarah Blyth Executive Director, Overdose Prevention Society

Dr. Neil Boyd Professor of Criminology, Simon Fraser University

Jennifer Breakspear Executive Director, Portland Hotel Society (PHS) Community Services Society

Chris Buchner Director of Communicable Diseases and Harm Reduction, Fraser Health

Judge Elisabeth Burgess Vancouver's Downtown Community Court

Dr. Richard Frank Professor of Health Economics, Harvard University

Len Garis Surrey Fire Chief

Mark Gervin Director of Legal Services, UBC's Indigenous Community Legal Clinic & Criminal Defence Lawyer

Yvette-Monique Gray Director of the Enforcement and Intelligence Division (Pacific Region), Canada Border Services Agency

Mario Harel President, Canadian Association of Chiefs of Police

Dr. Paul Hasselback Medical Health Officer, Central Vancouver Island

Dr. Bonnie Henry Chief Medical Officer, British Columbia

Dr. Ronald Joe Medical Director for Substance Use Services, Vancouver Coastal Health

Shelda Kastor Board Member and Secretary, Western Aboriginal Harm Reduction Society

Conor King Staff Sergeant, Victoria Police Department

David Lothian Chief of the Intelligence Section (Pacific Region), Canada Border Services Agency

Linda Lupini Executive Vice President, BC Provincial Health Services Authority & BC Emergency Health Services

Dr. Scott MacDonald Physician Lead, Crosstown Clinic

Leslie McBain Co-founder, Moms Stop the Harm

Dwayne McDonald Assistant Commissioner & Officer in Charge, RCMP Surrey Detachment

Dr. Shannon McDonald Acting Chief Medical Officer, First Nations Health Authority

Bill Mollard President, Union Gospel Mission

Clayton Pecknold Assistant Deputy Minister and Director of Police Services, Government of BC

Pivot Legal Society three representatives interviewed together

Laurence Rankin Deputy Chief Constable, Vancouver Police Department

Darrell Reid Vancouver Fire Chief

Mike Serr Deputy Chief, Abbotsford, BC, and Chair, Canadian Association of Chiefs of Police Drug Advisory Committee

Carolyn Sinclair Manager, BC Provincial Overdose Mobile Response Team

Marshall Smith Senior Advisor for Recovery Initiatives, British Columbia Centre on Substance Use & Chair, British Columbia Recovery Council

Bill Spearn Inspector, Vancouver Police Department

Dr. Mark Tyndall Executive Director, BC Centre for Disease Control

Andy Watson Strategic Communications Manager, BC Coroners Service

Jordan Westfall President, Canadian Association of People Who Use Drugs

Bonnie Wilson Operations Director (Inner-City Eastside) and Co-program Lead for Mental Health and Substance Use, Vancouver Coastal Health

Dr. Evan Wood Executive Director, BC Centre on Substance Use

NOTES

Chapter 1—What Is the Opioid Crisis?

8   **a record-shattering 13,913 people across Canada** Special Advisory Committee on the Epidemic of Opioid Overdoses, *National Report: Opioid-related Harms in Canada* (December 2019), https://health-infobase.canada.ca/substance-related-harms/opioids.

8   **the leading cause of death for 30- to 39-year-olds** Leslie Young, "Nearly 4,000 Canadians Died of Opioid Overdoses in 2017, a New Record," Global News, June 20, 2018, https://globalnews.ca/news/4282699/canada-opioid-death-statistics-2017.

9   **By 2018 that number had almost tripled, reaching 1542** BC Coroners Service, "Illicit Drug Toxicity Deaths in BC (January 1, 2009–October 31, 2019)" at 3, https://www2.gov.bc.ca/assets/gov/birth-adoption-death-marriage-and-divorce/deaths/coroners-service/statistical/illicit-drug.pdf.

10   **"We are in urgent need of temporary body storage"** Email correspondence from Aaron Burns, "BC Coroners Service: Body Storage (Vancouver and Area)" (December 19, 2016), released under the Freedom of Information and Protection of Privacy Act (File No. OCC-2018-83144) on June 4, 2018.

10 **"Bodies are kept at hospital morgues or funeral homes"** Ibid.

12 **In 2017, an estimated 70,237 people died from illicit drug overdoses in the U.S.** National Institute on Drug Abuse, "Overdose Death Rates" (revised January 2019), www.drugabuse.gov/related -topics/trends-statistics/overdose-death-rates.

12 **President Donald Trump has instead insisted on building a wall** Josh Katz, "How a Police Chief, a Governor and a Sociologist Would Spend $100 Billion to Solve the Opioid Crisis," *The New York Times* (February 14, 2018).

13 **illicit drug overdose deaths where fentanyl has been detected** BC Coroners Service, "Fentanyl-Detected Illicit Drug Overdose Deaths (January 1, 2012 to January 31, 2019)," www2.gov.bc.ca/assets/gov /birth-adoption-death-marriage-and-divorce/deaths/coroners-service /statistical/fentanyl-detected-overdose.pdf.

Chapter 2—Why Is Fentanyl Killing So Many People?

17 **Dr. Jules Blanchette, a 36-year-old veterinary surgeon, sold Inovar-Vet** *R. c. Blanchette*, [1990] J.Q. no 236 (C.A.Q.).

18 **The first time fentanyl is mentioned** *R. v. Reid*, 2008 NSPC 41, [2008] N.S.J. No. 287, para. 15.

18 **in just 10 months carfentanyl was detected** BC Coroners Service, "Fentanyl-Detected Illicit Drug Overdose Deaths (January 1, 2012 to March 31, 2018)," www2.gov.bc.ca/assets/gov/public-safety-and -emergency-services/death-investigation/statistical/fentanyl-detected -overdose.pdf.

21 **Purdue Pharma introduced OxyContin in the mid-1990s** Caitlin Esch, "How One Sentence Helped Set Off the Opioid Crisis," *Marketplace*, December 13, 2017, www.marketplace.org/2017/12/13 /health-care/uncertain-hour/opioid.

21 **Medical residents were allegedly taught** Jon Kelvey, "How
Advertising Shaped the First Opioid Epidemic: And What It Can
Teach Us About the Second," *Smithsonian Magazine*, April 3, 2018,
www.smithsonianmag.com/science-nature/how-advertising-shaped
-first-opioid-epidemic-180968444.

21 **The company has denied deceptive marketing** Harriet Jones,
"Purdue Pharma to End Marketing of Oxycontin," *WNPR*, February 12,
2018, http://wnpr.org/post/purdue-pharma-end-marketing-oxycontin.

22 **Some people have even chewed used fentanyl patches** *R. v. Chivers*,
2017 ONCJ 904, [2017] O.J. No. 6889, para. 6.

22 **Prescription drug theft has been increasing in provinces like
Ontario** Tara Carman & Vik Adhopia, "More Than Half a Million
Prescription Drugs Are Stolen Each Year—And Most Are Opioids,"
CBC News, June 27, 2018, www.cbc.ca/news/canada/missing-drugs
-pharmacies-part1-1.4708041.

22 **Some pointed to a study by the BC Coroners Service** BC Coroners
Service, "Preventing Pharmaceutical Opioid-Associated Mortality in
British Columbia: A Review of Prescribed Opioid Overdose Deaths,
2009–2013" (July 17, 2017), www2.gov.bc.ca/assets/gov/public-safety
-and-emergency-services/death-investigation/statistical/pharmaceutical
-opioid-mortality.pdf.

23 **On the morning of April 20, 2018, his parents found him in
his bedroom** Cindy E. Harnett, "Parents Called 911 and Injected
Naloxone, but It Was Too Late to Save Teen," *Times Colonist*
(Victoria), April 25, 2018.

24 **Preliminary data from a study by the BC Centre for Disease
Control** BC Centre for Disease Control, "BCCDC Public Knowledge
Summary: Analyzing Prescription Drug Histories Among People
Who Overdose" (February 21, 2018).

Chapter 3—Why Do People Start Using? Why Can't They Stop?

27 **"I help them decrease stress and anxiety"** Michael Stone, "My Story," https://michaelstoneteaching.com/my-story.

28 **"Unbeknownst to everybody, he was growing more desperate."** Carina Stone, Erin Robinsong, & Rose Riccio, "Michael Stone's Passing—Official Statement," https://michaelstoneteaching.com /official-statement-michael-stones-passing/#.

28 **he'd died of acute fentanyl toxicity** BC Coroners Service, "Coroner's Report into the Death of Stone, Michael Jason," Case No. 2017-1037-0048 (April 10, 2018).

29 **In BC, the vast majority of illicit drug overdose deaths are men** BC Coroners Service, "Illicit Drug Overdose Deaths in BC (January 1, 2008–March 31, 2018)," www2.gov.bc.ca/assets/gov/public-safety-and -emergency-services/death-investigation/statistical/illicit-drug.pdf.

29 **it wasn't possible to determine the frequency of drug use** Michael Egilson, *BC Coroners Service Death Review Panel: A Review of Illicit Drug Overdoses* (April 5, 2018) at 15 [*Death Review Panel*].

30 **only 9% of illicit drug overdose deaths were officially homeless people** Ibid. at 14.

30 **In BC in 2017, 59% of illicit drug overdose deaths occurred in private residences** BC Coroners Service, "Illicit Drug Overdose Deaths in BC (January 1, 2008–March 31, 2018)" at 12, www2.gov.bc.ca/assets /gov/public-safety-and-emergency-services/death-investigation /statistical/illicit-drug.pdf.

30 **More than half (52%) of illicit drug overdose deaths involved people using alone** *Death Review Panel* at 16.

31 **Two other reasons focus groups have found** Ibid. at 16.

34 **"Each of the friends used the drugs from the same delivery."** BC Coroners Service, "Coroner's Report into the Death of Adkin, Edmond Paul," Case No. 2016-0573-0157 (April 12, 2018).

35 **"Rarely did you see Paul without a smile"** Dignity Memorial, "Obituary: Edmond 'Paul' Adkin," www.dignitymemorial.com/en-ca /obituaries/kamloops-bc/edmond-adkin-7115359.

37 **Each ACE point represents a two- to fourfold increase** S.R. Dube, V.J. Felitti, M. Dong, D.P. Chapman, W.H. Giles, & R.F. Anda, "Childhood Abuse, Neglect and Household Dysfunction and the Risk of Illicit Drug Use: The Adverse Childhood Experience Study" (2003) 111(3) *Pediatrics* 564–572.

41 **classified as a mental disorder by the American Psychiatric Association** American Psychiatric Association, *Diagnostic and Statistical Manual of Mental Disorders*, 5th ed. (Washington, DC: American Psychiatric Publishing, 2013) ("DSM-5") at 541–546.

44 **"clinically significant distress or impairment in social, occupational, or other important areas of functioning"** Ibid. at 548.

44 **"escalating pattern in which an opioid is used to reduce withdrawal symptoms"** Ibid. at 549.

47 **Some studies have found that one in five lawyers experience** Indra Cidambi, "Drug and Alcohol Abuse in the Legal Profession," *Psychology Today* (July 17, 2017), www.psychologytoday.com/us/blog /sure-recovery/201707/drug-and-alcohol-abuse-in-the-legal-profession.

Chapter 4—Has Criminalizing Drugs Failed?

49 **for every mile of track laid through the Rocky Mountains** *Chinese Regulation Act, 1884*, 47 Vict., c. 4, s. 18 (Source: University of British Columbia. Library. Rare Books and Special Collections. The Chung Collection. CC-TX-279-14); CBC, "Legacy of Hate: Chinese Immigrants Encounter Prejudice and Violence as They Settled in Canada," www. cbc.ca/history/EPISCONTENTSE1EP11CH3PA3LE.html.

49 **Except for medical or surgical purposes, its use was punishable** *Extract from Votes and Proceedings of the Legislative Assembly, 25th*

February, 1885 (Source: University of British Columbia. Library. Rare Books and Special Collections. The Chung Collection. CC-TX-100-43-9).

50 **After the Chinese Regulation Act and other anti-Chinese laws**. Ibid.

50 **"Of course we ought to exclude them,"** House of Commons Debates, 5th Parl., 3rd Sess., Vol. 2, p. 1588 (May 4, 1885) (Sir John A. Macdonald).

51 **If you look around the world you will see that the Aryan races** Ibid. at 1585.

51 **Twelve-foot-wide banners bore slogans that read** "Vancouver Was in the Throes of Serious Riot Saturday Night," *The Weekly News-Advertiser* (Vancouver), Vol. XXI, No. 2, September 10, 1907.

52 *Awful effects of Opium Habit.* Cited in W.L. Mackenzie King, *The Need for the Suppression on the Opium Traffic in Canada*, 7–8 Edward VII, Sessional Paper No. 36b (Ottawa: 1908) at 7–8.

52 **"Smoking opium was not considered to be physically harmful"** R. Solomon & M. Green, "The First Century: The History of Nonmedical Opiate Use and Control Policies in Canada, 1870–1970" (1982) 20:2 *UWO Law Review* 307–337 at 309.

52 **"This crusade succeeded because it was directed against Chinese opium smokers"** Ibid. at 308.

53 **Despite over a century of trying to eradicate illicit drugs** Channing May, *Transnational Crime and the Developing World* (Global Financial Integrity: March 2017) at xi.

54 **From 1990 to 2007, the average price of heroin in the United States** Researchers adjusted prices for inflation and relative purity. See Dan Werb et al., "The Temporal Relationship Between Drug Supply Indicators: An Audit of International Government Surveillance Systems," *BMJ Open* 2013;3:e003077.

54 **Downward price trends were also observed in Europe and Australia** Ibid.

55 **during the Prohibition period, the potency of alcohol products increased by 150%** Leo Beletsky & Corey S. Davis, "Today's Fentanyl Crisis: Prohibition's Iron Law, Revised" (2017) 46 *International Journal of Drug Policy* 156–159 at 157.

55 **Richard Cowan, a Republican-turned-cannabis-activist** Richard C. Cowan, "How the Narcs Created Crack: A War Against Ourselves" 38(23) *National Review* 26–31 (December 5, 1986) at 27.

56 **Between 2008 and 2015, enforcement at the border with Mexico** Leo Beletsky & Corey S. Davis, "Today's Fentanyl Crisis: Prohibition's Iron Law, Revised" (2017) 46 *International Journal of Drug Policy* 156–159 at 157.

Chapter 5—Why Are Dealers Killing Their Customers?

57 **"I'm french speaking organic chemist so excuse my rusty english"** Siegfried, "Synthesis of Fentanyl" (undated), https://erowid.org/archive/rhodium/chemistry/fentanyl.html.

57 **The United Nations Office on Drugs and Crime's 2017 report** United Nations Office on Drugs and Crime, "Fentanyl and its Analogues—50 Years On" *Global Smart Update Volume 17* at 7.

58 **Dr. Mayer was able to obtain the necessary ingredients** Brian P. Mayer et al., "Chemical Attribution of Fentanyl Using Multivariate Statistical Analysis of Orthogonal Mass Spectral Data" (2016) 88 *Analytical Chemistry* 4303–4310 at 4305.

60 **99% pure illicit fentanyl can be bought from China** U.S. Drug Enforcement Administration, *2017 National Drug Threat Assessment* (October 2017) at 62, www.dea.gov/docs/DIR-040-17_2017-NDTA.pdf.

60 **Heroin in the Vancouver area typically sells for approximately $70,000 per kilogram** *R. v. Mann*, [2017] B.C.J. No. 2663, 2017 BCPC 401, para. 26.

62 **drug trafficking over the dark web is on the rise** United Nations Office on Drugs and Crime, "Global Overview of Drug Demand and

Supply: Latest Trends, Cross-Cutting Issues," *World Drug Report 2017* (Vienna: UN, 2017) at 42–46.

63 **some illicit fentanyl manufacturers in China were once offering customers free replacements** Eric Stewart, "Fentanyl," Vol. 79, No. 1—Just the Facts (RCMP: January 13, 2017).

Chapter 6—Can We Stop Fentanyl at Its Source?

66 **"We need to help [the media] by providing the right commentary"** Chad Skelton, "CBSA Spokeswoman Admits: We Tell Reporters 'Basically Nothing,'" *Vancouver Sun*, August 16, 2010.

73 **others are new "designer drugs" created by chemists working for the benefit of organized crime** United Nations Office on Drugs and Crime, "Fentanyl and Its Analogues—50 Years On" *Global Smart Update Volume 17* (Vienna: UNODC, 2017) at 4.

74 **Despite reportedly seizing 1.8 tonnes of illicit drugs between 2015 and 2017** "Thousands of Tons of Hallucinogens, Stimulants Busted in China," *The Standard* (Hong Kong), June 19, 2017.

74 **"My feeling is that it's just like a race and I will never catch up"** Nathan Vanderklippe, "China, Claiming Success on Fentanyl, Admits It Is Being Outrun by Criminal Chemists," *The Globe and Mail*, June 19, 2017.

74 **"Both Mexico and China are major source countries for fentanyl"** U.S. Drug Enforcement Administration, "FAQs-Fentanyl and Fentanyl-Related Substance," www.dea.gov/druginfo/fentanyl-faq.shtml.

77 **It turns out that under our federal postal legislation** Canada Post Corporation Act, R.S.C., 1985, c. C-10, s. 40(3). See *R. v Perkins*, 2018 BCSC 395. Some other judicial decisions have allowed controlled deliveries by the police without discussing the issue.

77 **cocaine, heroin, guns, grenades, stun guns, and even a rocket launcher** Canadian Association of Chiefs of Police, "Amendments to the *Canada Post Corporation Act*," Resolution #8—2015.

79 **They say that "micro-labs" could be in homes and apartments** RCMP, "Fentanyl Drug Labs: Awareness for Landlords and Rental Services," February 28, 2017, www.rcmp-grc.gc.ca/en/fentanyl-drug -labs-awareness-landlords-and-rental-services.

80 **It identified three cases of varying levels of sophistication** United Nations Office on Drugs and Crime, "Fentanyl and Its Analogues— 50 Years On," *Global Smart Update Volume* 17 at 7.

81 **Since fentanyl is a synthetic drug that can be made in a number of ways** Brian P. Mayer et al., "Chemical Attribution of Fentanyl Using Multivariate Statistical Analysis of Orthogonal Mass Spectral Data" (2016), 88 *Analytical Chemistry*, 4303–4310.

Chapter 7—Who's Been Hardest Hit?

84 **"Brandon had a smile that lit up a room"** Brandon Janson Foundation, "Brandon's Story," https://brandonjansenfoundation.com /brandons-story.

84 **"Brandon was an engaging young man who seemed motivated"** Michael Egilson, *Verdict at Coroners Inquest: Jansen, Brandon Juhani*, File no. 2016:1027:0004 (January 25, 2017).

87 **Egilson found that 18% of those who'd had a fatal illicit drug overdose** Michael Egilson, *BC Coroners Service Death Review Panel: A Review of Illicit Drug Overdoses* (April 5, 2018) at 19.

87 **a full 66% had been involved with BC Corrections** Ibid.

87 **The first two weeks after release are especially dangerous** Elizabeth L.C. Merrall et al., "Meta-Analysis of Drug-Related Deaths Soon After Release from Prison" (2010), 105 *Addiction*, 1545–1554.

88 **44% of those who fatally overdosed and had been in custody died** Michael Egilson, *BC Coroners Service Death Review Panel: A Review of Illicit Drug Overdoses* (April 5, 2018) at 19.

89 **It's not surprising that there are so many overdoses among people who are homeless** Ibid. at 14.

92 **compared with only 0.3% of non-Indigenous children** Statistics Canada, *Aboriginal Peoples in Canada: First Nations People, Métis and Inuit*, Catalogue no. 99-011-X2011001 (National Household Survey, 2011) at 5.

94 **Data from the First Nations Health Authority** First Nations Health Authority, *Overdose Data and First Nations in BC: Preliminary Findings* at 7.

95 **Compared with non-Indigenous women** Ibid.

Chapter 8—Can We Prosecute Our Way Out?

99 **"It was a dark and stormy night"** Bick's account of the facts of this case was corroborated with the audio-recording of the trial in *R. v. Bainbridge*. British Columbia Supreme Court (New Westminster), Courtroom #413, April 20, 2015 (Chilliwack Indictment #57723-2).

105 **an "exemplary sentence for an exemplary case"** *R. v. McCormick*, [2017] B.C.J. No. 171, 2017 BCPC 22, para. 7.

105 **"Mr. McCormick was the supplier to a mid-level drug trafficker"** Ibid., para. 64.

105 **"I recognize that a sentence above any established range"** Ibid., para. 85.

106 **"Recognizing a different and markedly higher sentencing range"** *R. v. Smith*, [2017] B.C.J. No. 471, 2017 BCCA 112, para. 49.

108 **"Addiction motivated nearly all the individuals who were engaging in street-level trafficking"** Haley Hrymak, "A Bad Deal: British Columbia's Emphasis on Deterrence and Increasing Prison Sentences for Street-Level Fentanyl Traffickers" (2018) 41:3 *Manitoba Law Journal* 149–179 at 158.

108 **"Research shows that the threat of an increased jail term does not dissolve an addiction"** Haley Hrymak, "Calling for Harm Reduction: The Opioid Crisis and What the Courts Can Do," *2018 UBC Interdisciplinary Legal Studies Graduate Conference* (Vancouver, BC: May 11, 2018). See also Caitlin Elizabeth Hughes & Alex Stevens, "What Can We Learn from the Portuguese Decriminalization of Illicit Drugs?" (2010) 50 *British Journal of Criminology* 999.

108 **"The VPD will not distinguish between the two"** Vancouver Police Department, *Vancouver Police Department Drug Policy* (adopted September 2006).

109 **Between 2015 and 2017, the VPD filed a total of 899 illicit drug trafficking charges** Vancouver Police Department—Organized Crime Section, "Trafficking/PPT Statistics & Heroin/Fentanyl Pricing" (May 3, 2018) (on file with author).

110 **Only 31 out of 899 (3.4%) of drug trafficking charges in Vancouver** Ibid.

110 **"Prison has been characterized by some as a finishing school for criminals"** *R. v. Proulx*, [2000] 1 S.C.R. 61, para. 16.

113 **Jordan was arrested in December 2008** *R. v. Jordan*, 2016 SCC 27, [2016] 1 S.C.R. 631, para. 9.

113 **"It 'rewards the wrong behaviour, frustrates the well-intentioned'"** Ibid., para. 40 (citations omitted).

114 **An alleged fentanyl dealer in Ontario recently had his charges stayed** *R. v. McCready*, [2017] O.J. No. 621, 2017 ONCJ 15.

116 **"More severe punishments do not 'chasten' individuals"** U.S. National Institute of Justice, "National Institute of Justice Five Things About Deterrence" (May 2016), www.ncjrs.gov/pdffiles1/nij/247350.pdf; see also, e.g., Heather Mann et al., "What Deters Crime? Comparing the Effectiveness of Legal, Social, and Internal Sanctions Across Countries" (2016) 7:85 *Frontiers in Psychology* 1–13

at 2; Daniel S. Nagin, "Deterrence in the Twenty-First Century," in M. Tonry, ed., *Crime and Justice in America: 1975–2025* (Chicago: University of Chicago Press, 2013) 199–264.

116 **legal sanctions also have less of a deterrent effect on serious offences** Heather Mann et al., "What Deters Crime? Comparing the Effectiveness of Legal, Social, and Internal Sanctions Across Countries" (2016) 7:85 *Frontiers in Psychology* 1–13 at 2.

116 **President Donald Trump has gone so far as to propose that fentanyl traffickers be subject to the death penalty** U.S. National Institute of Justice, "National Institute of Justice Five Things About Deterrence" (May 2016), www.ncjrs.gov/pdffiles1/nij/247350.pdf.

117 **"Specifically, annual street-level data suggest the price of heroin, cocaine, crack cocaine"** BC Centre for Excellence in HIV/AIDS, "Drug Situation in Vancouver" (October 2009) at 9.

Chapter 9—What Is Naloxone and Is It the Solution?

123 **"They call me 'Little Doug' on the street"** Toward the Heart, "In Memorial: Douglas Nickerson ('Little Doug')," https://vimeo.com /244131663.

125 **studies have shown naloxone to be 94% effective when administered by laypeople** Michael A. Irvine et al., "Distribution of Take-Home Opioid Antagonist Kits During a Synthetic Opioid Epidemic in British Columbia, Canada: A Modelling Study" (2018) *The Lancet Public Health*, http://dx.doi.org/10.1016/S2468-2667(18)30044-6 at 2.

127 **Between January and October 2016, 298 deaths were averted** BC Centre for Disease Control, "Study: Wide Distribution of Naloxone Can Slash Overdose Deaths During Epidemics" (April 18, 2018), www.bccdc.ca/about/news-stories/news-releases/2017/take-home -naloxone; see Michael A. Irvine et al., "Distribution of Take-Home Opioid Antagonist Kits During a Synthetic Opioid Epidemic in

British Columbia, Canada: A Modelling Study" (2018) *The Lancet Public Health,* http://dx.doi.org/10.1016/S2468-2667(18)30044-6.

130 **"Naloxone should be readily available to all Canadians at no cost"** Canadian Pharmacists Association, "Environmental Scan: Access to Naloxone Across Canada" (November 2017) at 3, www.pharmacists.ca /cpha-ca/assets/File/cpha-on-the-issues/Environmental%20Scan%20 -%20Access%20to%20Naloxone%20Across%20Canada_Final.pdf.

130 **A recent death review panel by the BC Coroners Service** Michael Egilson, *BC Coroners Service Death Review Panel: A Review of Illicit Drug Overdoses* (April 5, 2018) at 4.

130 **A program in the United Kingdom that gives prisoners these kits** European Monitoring Centre for Drugs and Drug Addiction, *European Drug Report 2017: Trends and Developments* (EMCDAA: Belgium, 2017) at 79.

130 **The coroner's inquest jury recommended that all substance use treatment centres** Michael Egilson, *Verdict at Coroners Inquest: Jansen, Brandon Juhani,* File no. 2016:1027:0004 (January 25, 2017).

131 **"Naloxone does not truly save lives, it merely extends them"** Kevin Miller, "LePage Vetoes Bill Aimed at Increasing Access to Overdose Antidote," *Press Herald,* April 20, 2016.

131 **delaying the rapid distribution of take-home naloxone costs lives** Michael A. Irvine et al., "Distribution of Take-Home Opioid Antagonist Kits During a Synthetic Opioid Epidemic in British Columbia, Canada: A Modelling Study" (2018) *The Lancet Public Health,* http://dx.doi.org/10.1016/S2468-2667(18)30044-6.

131 **intravenous drug users who were educated and trained in how to respond to an overdose** Karen H. Seal et al., "Naloxone Distribution and Cardiopulmonary Resuscitation Training for Injection Drug Users to Prevent Heroin Overdose Death: A Pilot Intervention Study" (2005) 82:2 *Journal of Urban Health: Bulletin of the New York*

Academy of Medicine 303–311; see also Alexander R. Bazazi et al., "Preventing Opiate Overdose Deaths: Examining Objections to Take-Home Naloxone" (2010) 21(4) *Journal of Health Care for the Poor and Underserved* 1108–1113.

131 **"opioid overdose education may reduce incremental risky behaviors"** Todd Kerensky & Alexander Y. Walley, "Opioid Overdose Prevention and Naloxone Rescue Kits: What We Know and What We Don't Know" (2017) 12:4 *Addiction Science & Clinical Practice* 1–7 at 3.

132 **"Be Prepared. Get Naloxone. Save a Life."** U.S. Surgeon General, "Surgeon General's Advisory on Naloxone and Opioid Overdose," www.surgeongeneral.gov/priorities/opioid-overdose-prevention/naloxone-advisory.html.

133 **"Addiction doesn't need to be a death sentence."** PHS Community Service Society, "Insite Supervised Injection Facility," www.phs.ca/project/insite-supervised-injection-facility.

133 **Studies have found that bystanders often don't call 911** See Kathryn Hawk & Gail D'Onofrio, "Reducing Fatal Opioid Overdose: Prevention, Treatment and Harm Reduction Strategies" (2015) 88 *Yale Journal of Biology and Medicine* 235–245 at 241–242.

133 **Research has shown that drug overdose Good Samaritan laws** Ibid.

138 **BC's Take Home Naloxone program estimates** Toward the Heart, "THN in BC Infograph" (updated May 15, 2018), http://towardtheheart.com/thn-in-bc-infograph.

Chapter 10—Don't Supervised Injection Sites Enable Drug Use?

145 **And there have been *zero* deaths** Overdose Prevention Society, *2017 Year End Report* at 2, 4.

146 **Blyth shared a couple of the comments she's received from clients and peers** Ibid. at 7–11.

148 **There has yet to be a single documented fatal overdose** Chloé Potier, Vincent Laprévote, Françoise Dubois-Arber, Olivier Cottencin, & Benjamin Rolland, "Supervised Injection Services: What Has Been Demonstrated? A Systematic Literature Review" (2014) 145 *Drug & Alcohol Dependence* 48–68 at 62; Harm Reduction Coalition, *Alternatives to Public Injecting* (2016) at 15, http://harmreduction.org/wp-content /uploads/2016/05/Alternatives-to-Public-Injection-report.pdf.

148 **Not a single person died** Vancouver Coastal Health, "Insite User Statistics," www.vch.ca/public-health/harm-reduction/supervised -consumption-sites/insite-user-statistics.

148 **In 2017, that had risen to six overdoses every day** Ibid.

148 **Vancouver's overdose prevention sites reversed 1225 overdoses** Vancouver Coastal Health, "Overdose statistics—November 2017" (December 20, 2017), www.vch.ca/about-us/news/overdose-statistics -november-2017.

148 **in Vancouver one person died from an illicit drug overdose every day in 2017** BC Coroners Service, "Illicit Drug Overdose Deaths in BC (January 1, 2018–March 31, 2018)," www2.gov.bc.ca/assets/gov /public-safety-and-emergency-services/death-investigation/statistical /illicit-drug.pdf.

149 **"There has been no discernible negative impact on the public safety"** *Canada (Attorney General) v. PHS Community Services Society*, [2011] 3 SCR 134, para. 133.

149 **These studies found no evidence of negative impacts** See Urban Research Initiative of the British Columbia Centre for Excellence in HIV/AIDS, *Finding from the Evaluation of Vancouver's Pilot Medically Supervised Safer Injecting Facility—Insite* (June 2009); E. Wood, M.W. Tyndall, J.S. Montaner, & T. Kerr, "Summary of Findings from the Evaluation of a Pilot Medically Supervised Safer Injecting Facility" (2006) 175(11) *Canadian Medical Association Journal* 1399–1404.

149 **A study in** *The Lancet* **found that after intravenous drug users started using Insite** T. Kerr, M.K. Tyndall, K. Li, J. Montaner, & E. Wood, "Safer Injection Facility Use and Syringe Sharing in Injection Drug Users" (2005) 366(9482) *Lancet* 316–318.

149 **In 2017, Insite provided 3708 such clinical treatments** Vancouver Coastal Health, "Insite User Statistics," www.vch.ca/public-health /harm-reduction/supervised-consumption-sites/insite-user-statistics.

150 **433 clients went to Onsite and had an average stay of 11 days** Ibid.

150 **"supervised injection facilities are unlikely to result in reduced use of addiction-treatment services"** E. Wood, M.W. Tyndall, R. Zhang, J. Stoltz, C. Lai, J.S.G. Montaner, & T. Kerr, "Attendance at Supervised Injecting Facilities and Use of Detoxification Services" (2006) 354(23) *New England Journal of Medicine* 2512–2514 at 2513.

151 **Researchers found "significant reductions in public injection drug use"** E. Wood, T. Kerr, W. Small, K. Li, D. Marsh, J.S. Montaner, & M.W. Tyndall, "Changes in Public Order After the Opening of a Medically Supervised Safer Injecting Facility for Illicit Injection Drug Users" (2004) 171(7) *Canadian Medical Association Journal* 731–734 at 733.

151 **But there was a drop in vehicle thefts and break-ins** E. Wood, M.W. Tyndall, C. Lai, J.S.G. Montaner, & T. Kerr, "Impact of a Medically Supervised Safer Injecting Facility on Drug Dealing and Other Drug-Related Crime" (2006) 1(1) *Substance Abuse Treatment, Prevention, and Policy* 13.

151 **Researchers saw this as doubly beneficial** K. DeBeck, E. Wood, R. Zhang, M. Tyndall, J. Montaner, & T. Kerr, "Police and Public Health Partnerships: Evidence from the Evaluation of Vancouver's Supervised Injection Facility" (2008) 3(1) *Substance Abuse Treatment, Prevention, and Policy* 11.

151 **Medical research has also found that supervised consumption sites** T. Kerr, M.W. Tyndall, C. Lai, J.S.G. Montaner, & E. Wood, "Drug-Related Overdoses within a Medically Supervised Safer

Injection Facility"(2006) 17(5) *International Journal of Drug Policy* 436–441.

152 **"I'm dead against that."** The Canadian Press, "Doug Ford Says He's 'Dead Against' Supervised Injection Sites," CBC News, April 20, 2018, www.cbc.ca/news/canada/windsor/doug-ford-says-he-s-dead-against -supervised-injection-sites-1.4628547.

152 **"helping addicts inject poison into their bodies is not a solution"** Tim Kalinowski, "Kenney Opposes Consumption Sites," *Lethbridge Herald*, March 1, 2018, http://lethbridgeherald.com/news/lethbridge -news/2018/03/01/kenney-opposes-consumption-sites.

152 **"Why isn't the federal government massively increasing resources for the Canada Border Services Agency"** Jason Kenney (@jkenney verified account), Twitter, March 2, 2018, at 11:19 a.m.

152 **"SIFs [safe injection facilities] are counterproductive and danger- ous"** U.S. Attorney's Office for the District of Vermont, "Statement of the U.S. Attorney's Office Concerning Proposed Injection Sites," Press Release, December 13, 2017, www.justice.gov/usao-vt/pr /statement-us-attorney-s-office-concerning-proposed-injection-sites.

153 **A study in the *American Journal of Public Health* found that "the average Insite user had been injecting for 16 years"** Urban Research Initiative of the British Columbia Centre for Excellence in HIV/AIDS, *Finding from the Evaluation of Vancouver's Pilot Medically Supervised Safer Injecting Facility—Insite* (June 2009); see T. Kerr, M. Tyndall, R. Zhang, C. Lai, J. Montaner, & E. Wood, "Circumstances of First Injection Among Illicit Drug Users Accessing a Medically Supervised Safer Injection Facility" (2007) 97(7) *American Journal of Public Health* 1228–1230.

155 **police-reported crime has declined significantly since the early 1970s** Kathryn Keighley, "Police-Reported Crime Statistics in Canada, 2016" (Statistics Canada: July 24, 2017), www150.statcan.gc.ca/n1/en /pub/85-002-x/2017001/article/54842-eng.pdf?st=UOEV3Typ.

159   **Preliminary data from Insite suggests that while regular opioid users don't tend to dispose of drugs** BC Centre on Substance Use, *Drug Checking as a Harm Reduction Intervention: Evidence Review Report* (December 2017) at 21.

161   **A review of published research by the BC Centre on Substance Use** Ibid. at 22.

Chapter 11—Is Providing "Safe Drugs" Giving Up On People?

165   **The results of the NAOMI study were published in the *New England Journal of Medicine* in August 2009** Eugenia Oviedo-Joekes et al., "Diacetylmorphine versus Methadone for the Treatment of Opioid Addiction" (2009) 361 *New England Journal of Medicine* 777–786. All statistics provided about the NAOMI study are from this article.

167   **The findings from the SALOME study were published in the *Journal of the American Medical Association Psychiatry*** Eugenia Oviedo-Joekes et al., "Hydromorphone Compared with Diacetylmorphine for Long-Term Opioid Dependence: A Randomized Clinical Trial" (2016) 73(5) *JAMA Psychiatry* 447–455.

168   **"Our policy is to take heroin out of the hands of addicts, not to put it into their arms"** *Providence Health Care Society v. Canada (Attorney General)*, 2014 BCSC 936, para. 21; see also Laura Eggertson, "Health Minister Ends Special Access to Prescription Heroin," *CMAJ*, November 19, 2013 185 (17) E773–E774.

168   **"I was shocked to learn today that Health Canada approved applications to give heroin to addicts"** Peter O'Neil, "Ottawa Overrules Health Officials on Vancouver Heroin Replacement Study," *Vancouver Sun*, October 4, 2013.

168   **"It was a life of hell," he said** James Keller, "B.C. Health Provider and Patients File Lawsuit Over Prescription Heroin Access," *Vancouver Sun*, November 13, 2013.

168 **Love returned to illicit heroin** *Providence Health Care Society v. Canada (Attorney General)*, 2014 BCSC 936, para. 59.

170 **A major study of the economic implications of these medications** Nick Bansback et al., "Cost-Effectiveness of Hydromorphone for Severe Opioid Use Disorder: Findings from the SALOME Randomized Clinical Trial" (2018) 113 *Addiction* 1264–1273 at 1271.

170 **"It is the application of a 'bundle' of interventions"** *Providence Health Care Society v. Canada (Attorney General)*, 2014 BCSC 936, para. 26.

171 **It's prescribed for opioid use disorder in the United Kingdom, Switzerland, Germany, Denmark, and the Netherlands** BC Ministry of Health and BC Centre on Substance Use, *Guidance for Injectable Opioid Agonist Treatment for Opioid Use Disorder* (2017) at 15, www.bccsu.ca/wp-content/uploads/2017/10/BC-iOAT-Guidelines-10 .2017.pdf.

175 **"The goal of this recommendation is to give addicted persons a 'clean opioid'"** Vancouver Police Department, *The Opioid Crisis: The Need for Treatment on Demand: Review and Recommendations* (May 2017) at 22, http://vancouver.ca/police/assets/pdf/reports-policies/opioid -crisis.pdf.

Chapter 12—How Can We Help People Stop Using?

181 *British Medical Journal* **which found that "patients who 'success- fully' completed inpatient detoxification"** John Strang et al., "Loss of Tolerance and Overdose Mortality After Inpatient Opiate Detoxification: Follow Up Study" (2003) *BMJ* May 3; 326(7396): 959–960.

181 **"this approach has been associated with elevated risk of HIV and hepatitis C transmission"** BC Ministry of Health and BC Centre on Substance Use, *A Guideline for the Clinical Management of Opioid Use Disorder* (June 5, 2017) at 11, www.bccsu.ca/wp-content/uploads/2017 /06/BC-OUD-Guidelines_June2017.pdf.

182 **In fact, relapse rates are 60% to 90%** Julie Bruneau et al., "Management of Opioid Use Disorders: A National Clinical Practice Guideline," *CMAJ* 2018 March 5; 190:E247-57 at E253-4.

184 **2017 Vancouver Police Department report on the opioid crisis** Vancouver Police Department, *The Opioid Crisis: The Need for Treatment on Demand: Review and Recommendations* (May 2017) at 25, http://vancouver.ca/police/assets/pdf/reports-policies/opioid -crisis.pdf.

184 **New national guidelines for treating opioid use disorder were published in the *Canadian Medical Association Journal* in March 2018** Julie Bruneau et al., "Management of Opioid Use Disorders: A National Clinical Practice Guideline," *CMAJ* (March 5, 2018), 190:E2 47–57; see also Centre for Addiction and Mental Health, "Opioid Agonist Therapy" (2016), www.camh.ca/-/media/files/oat-info-for -clients.pdf.

187 **"there are increased odds of success when doses are reduced gradually"** BC Ministry of Health and BC Centre on Substance Use, "A Guideline for the Clinical Management of Opioid Use Disorder" (June 5, 2017) at 30, www.bccsu.ca/wp-content/uploads/2017/06/BC -OUD-Guidelines_June2017.pdf.

187 **These first-line treatments just aren't effective for approximately 10% of people with opioid use disorder** Providence Health Care, "About SALOME," www.providencehealthcare.org/salome/about -us.html.

187 **more than half of those who start treatment with Suboxone or methadone discontinue it** BC Ministry of Health and BC Centre on Substance Use, *Guidance for Injectable Opioid Agonist Treatment for Opioid Use Disorder* (2017) at 14, www.bccsu.ca/wp-content/uploads /2017/10/BC-iOAT-Guidelines-10.2017.pdf.

187 **new guidelines for opioid use disorder say that residential treat-ment and psychosocial treatment** Julie Bruneau et al.,

"Management of Opioid Use Disorders: A National Clinical Practice Guideline," *CMAJ* (March 5, 2018), 190:E247-57 at E253; BC Ministry of Health and BC Centre on Substance Use, *A Guideline for the Clinical Management of Opioid Use Disorder* (June 5, 2017) at 31, www.bccsu.ca /wp-content/uploads/2017/06/BC-OUD-Guidelines_June2017.pdf.

188 **Controversially, a significant majority of Canadians recently polled** Angus Reid, "Opioids in Canada: One in Eight Have Family or Close Friends Who Faced Addiction," January 11, 2018, http://angusreid.org /opioid-crisis.

188 **U.S. National Institute of Drug Abuse estimates that every $1 spent on addiction treatment** National Institute on Drug Abuse, *Principles of Drug Addiction Treatment: A Research-Based Guide*, 3rd ed. (January 2018) at 14.

Chapter 13—Won't Decriminalization Make Things Worse?

193 **I never once saw Jim smile** Jim is a pseudonym.

197 **A stunning 70% of federal offenders are admitted to prison** Fraser McVie, "Drugs in Federal Corrections—The Issues and Challenges" (undated), www.csc-scc.gc.ca/research/forum/e133/e133c-eng.shtml.

197 **Sociologists believe that stigma flows from three main sources** Robin Room, "Stigma, Social Inequality and Alcohol and Drug Use" (2005) 24 *Drug and Alcohol Review* 143–155 at 147, 149.

197 **the Supreme Court of Canada has recognized that all criminal offences generate stigma** *R. v. Creighton*, [1993] 3 S.C.R. 3, para. 21.

199 **"You must not possess drug paraphernalia"** BC Provincial Court, "Probation Pick List" (May 1, 2017) at 14.

200 **The only reason they require Health Canada approval is the existence of the drug possession offence** *Canada (Attorney General) v. PHS Community Services Society*, [2011] 3 SCR 134, 2011 SCC 44 at paras. 19, 20, and 109.

202 **Property theft typically generates a 10 to 20% return** Eric Stewart, "Fentanyl," Vol. 79, No. 1—Just the Facts (Ottawa: RCMP, January 13, 2017), www.rcmp-grc.gc.ca/en/gazette/fentanyl?fent.

203 **"For opioid dependent inmates released from a correctional facility"** Michael Egilson, *Verdict at Coroners Inquest: Jansen, Brandon Juhani*, File no. 2016:1027:0004 (January 25, 2017) at 5.

208 **Experts at the UNODC concluded that the "range of drugs and drug markets"** United Nations Office on Drugs and Crime, *Executive Summary: Conclusions and Policy Recommendations* (Vienna: UN, 2018) at 1, www.unodc.org/wdr2018/prelaunch/WDR18_Booklet_1_EXSUM.pdf.

209 **It costs taxpayers $116,000 a year to keep someone in federal prison in Canada** Correctional Service Canada, "CSC Statistics—Key Facts and Figures" (June 2017), www.csc-scc.gc.ca/publications/005007-3024 -eng.shtml.

209 **half of all federal inmates are imprisoned on drug-related charges** E. Ann Carson, "Prisoners in 2016" (U.S. Department of Justice, Bureau of Justice Statistics: January 2018) at 1, www.bjs.gov/content /pub/pdf/p16.pdf.

209 **fewer than one in six people with drug use disorders are receiving treatment** Ibid.

211 **Illicit drug manufacturing and drug trafficking remain crimes** Caitlin Elizabeth Hughes & Alex Stevens, "What Can We Learn from the Portuguese Decriminalization of Illicit Drugs?" (2010) 50 *British Journal of Criminology* 999 at 1001–1002.

211 **written by an American constitutional lawyer and published by the CATO Institute** Glenn Greenwald, *Drug Decriminalization in Portugal: Lessons for Creating Fair and Successful Drug Policies* (Washington, DC: CATO Institute, 2009).

212 **Portugal "may offer a model for other nations"** Caitlin Elizabeth Hughes & Alex Stevens, "What Can We Learn from the Portuguese

Decriminalization of Illicit Drugs?" (2010) 50 *British Journal of Criminology* 999–1022 at 1018.

212 **best available data from the National Statistics Institute in Portugal reveals a massive drop** Caitlin Elizabeth Hughes & Alex Stevens, "A Resounding Success or a Disastrous Failure: Re-Examining the Interpretation of Evidence on the Portuguese Decriminalisation of Illicit Drugs." (2012) 31 *Drug and Alcohol Review* 101–113 at 105–108.

212 **"It may also be another indicator of falling levels of heroin use"** Caitlin Elizabeth Hughes & Alex Stevens, *The Effects of the Decriminalization of Drug Use in Portugal* (Oxford, The Beckley Foundation, 2007) at 3 (citations omitted).

213 **Overall, these mixed results are seen as a net benefit** Caitlin Elizabeth Hughes & Alex Stevens, "A Resounding Success or a Disastrous Failure: Re-Examining the Interpretation of Evidence on the Portuguese Decriminalisation of Illicit Drugs." (2012) 31 *Drug and Alcohol Review* 101–113 at 105.

213 **By 2005, 65% of people were referred for cannabis, 15% for heroin** Caitlin Elizabeth Hughes & Alex Stevens, *The Effects of the Decriminalization of Drug Use in Portugal* (Oxford, The Beckley Foundation, 2007) at 3.

216 **the equivalent of a fully-loaded large passenger aircraft crashing and killing everyone aboard** Adam Miller, "Why the Opioid Crisis Isn't a Bigger Federal Election Issue", CBC, October 5, 2019, https://www.cbc.ca/news/health/opioid-crisis-election-1.5309759.

Chapter 14—How Can We Solve This Crisis?

222 **prohibition has left the drug market as a "free-for-all"** I have to give credit to Pivot Legal Society for making this point in my interview with them.

222   **Lisa Lapointe, chief coroner with the BC Coroners Service** Lisa Lapointe, "Scare Tactics Less Effective in Overdose Crisis," December 2, 2017, https://news.gov.bc.ca/factsheets/scare-tactics-less-effective -in-overdose-crisis.

224   **Research has found that having higher self-esteem** BC Government, "Talking to Youth," www2.gov.bc.ca/gov/content/overdose/talking -to-youth.

224   **tips from the experts about how to talk to youth about substance use** Ibid. Copyright © Province of British Columbia. All rights reserved. Reproduced with permission of the Province of British Columbia.

227   **It is important that help (9-1-1) is called immediately in the event of an overdose** BC Provincial Health Services, BC Centre for Disease Control and TowardtheHeart.com, *Fentanyl-Induced Muscle Rigidity* (July 24, 2017) at 2.

231   **"Human beings have long looked to faith for strength and support"** Alexandre Laudet et al., "The Role of Social Supports, Spirituality, Religiousness, Life Meaning and Affiliation with 12-Step Fellowships in Quality of Life Satisfaction Among Individuals in Recovery from Alcohol and Drug Problems" (2006) *Alcohol Treat Quarterly* 24(1-2): 33–73.

231   **"substance users often come into recovery feeling abandoned by God"** Ibid.

232   **"In retrospect, I can see that God has been with me all the time"** Ibid.

232   **A study of 14 countries (including Canada) by the World Health Organization** Robin Room, "Stigma, Social Inequality and Alcohol and Drug Use" (2005) 24 *Drug and Alcohol Review* 143–155 at 145.

ACKNOWLEDGMENTS

Launching this project without any research team or funding was exciting, but daunting. We're in the midst of an international public health emergency, so I didn't want to waste any time. I'm very grateful for the support that quickly came in when I needed it from an individual donor, the Macdonald Laurier Institute for Public Policy, and the University of British Columbia, Peter A. Allard School of Law. My student research assistants, Emilly Porter, Matthew Scott, and Emily Chung, each made distinct contributions to this book, and I appreciate their hard work and passion for this topic. Haley Hrymak also provided valuable suggestions on the manuscript. I want to thank Lisa Godfrey for her timely, accurate, and diligent work transcribing all my research interviews. The City of Vancouver Archives, Vancouver Coastal Health Research Institute, Providence Healthcare, Fraser Health, and Island Health also need to be acknowledged for facilitating access to documentation and their experts.

I'm so happy to be publishing another book with the great team at Penguin Random House. I especially appreciated Diane Turbide's quick, enthusiastic response when I first pitched the project. Her great advice to me hadn't changed: make the issue real for people, don't just write a policy report. It was a pleasure working with Justin Stoller and Helen Smith on revising the manuscript. I really appreciated their ideas, challenges, and encouragement.

My biggest word of thanks is reserved for my wife, Claudia. One minute she's my editorial assistant and policy strategist, and the next my best friend and comforter. When I got on a writing streak, which could last for days at a time, she cleared the schedule and took care of all of life's important details so that I could get down on paper what was in my head.

Finally, I'd like to thank all the people I interviewed and got to know for this book. You are heroes, working in incredibly difficult circumstances, during a crisis you never asked for. Your dedication, professionalism, and championing of new ideas have saved lives. I hope that by sharing your stories and expertise many people will come to see, as I have, that what's needed most is understanding, care, and compassion.

INDEX